T0321084

SGLT-2 Inhibitors

Editors

RAGAVENDRA R. BALIGA
DEEPAK L. BHATT

HEART FAILURE CLINICS

www.heartfailure.theclinics.com

Consulting Editor
EDUARDO BOSSONE

Founding Editor
JAGAT NARULA

October 2022 • Volume 18 • Number 4

ELSEVIER

1600 John F. Kennedy Boulevard • Suite 1800 • Philadelphia, Pennsylvania, 19103-2899

http://www.theclinics.com

HEART FAILURE CLINICS Volume 18, Number 4
October 2022 ISSN 1551-7136, ISBN-13: 978-0-323-96046-5

Editor: Joanna Collett
Developmental Editor: Jessica Cañaberal

Heart Failure Clinics (ISSN 1551-7136) is published quarterly by Elsevier Inc., 360 Park Avenue South, New York, NY 10010-1710. Months of publication are January, April, July, and October. Business and editorial offices: 1600 John F. Kennedy Boulevard, Suite 1800, Philadelphia, PA 19103-2899. Periodicals postage paid at New York, NY, and additional mailing offices. Subscription prices are USD 277.00 per year for US individuals, USD 681.00 per year for US institutions, USD 100.00 per year for US students and residents, USD 300.00 per year for Canadian individuals, USD 701.00 per year for Canadian institutions, USD 315.00 per year for international individuals, USD 701.00 per year for international institutions, and USD 100.00 per year for Canadian and foreign students/residents. To receive student and resident rate, orders must be accompanied by name of affiliated institution, date of term, and the *signature* of program/residency coordinator on institution letterhead. Orders will be billed at individual rate until proof of status is received. Foreign air speed delivery is included in all *Clinics* subscription prices. All prices are subject to change without notice. **POSTMASTER:** Send address changes to *Heart Failure Clinics*, Elsevier Health Sciences Division, Subscription Customer Service, 3251 Riverport Lane, Maryland Heights, MO 63043. **Customer Service: 1-800-654-2452 (US and Canada). From outside of the US and Canada, call 314-447-8871. Fax: 314-447-8029. For print support, E-mail: JournalsCustomerService-usa@elsevier.com. For online support, E-mail: JournalsOnlineSupport-usa@elsevier.com.**

Reprints. For copies of 100 or more of articles in this publication, please contact the Commercial Reprints Department, Elsevier Inc., 360 Park Avenue South, New York, NY 10010-1710. Tel.: 212-633-3874; Fax: 212-633-3820; E-mail: reprints@elsevier.com.

Heart Failure Clinics is covered in *MEDLINE/PubMed (Index Medicus).*

Contributors

CONSULTING EDITOR

EDUARDO BOSSONE, MD, PhD, FCCP, FESC, FACC Consulting Editor, *Heart Failure Clinics*, Director, Division of Cardiology, AORN Antonio Cardarelli Hospital, Naples, Italy

EDITORS

RAGAVENDRA R. BALIGA, MD, MBA, FACP, FRCP (Edin), FACC
Inaugural Cardio-Oncologist Professor and Attending Cardiologist, Division of Cardiology, The Ohio State University Wexner Medical Center, Columbus, Ohio, USA

DEEPAK L. BHATT, MD, MPH, FACC, FAHA, FSCAI, FESC
Executive Director of Interventional Cardiovascular Programs, Brigham and Women's Hospital Heart & Vascular Center, Professor of Medicine, Harvard Medical School, Boston, Massachusetts, USA

EDUARDO BOSSONE, MD, PhD, FCCP, FESC, FACC
Consulting Editor, *Heart Failure Clinics*, Director, Division of Cardiology, AORN Antonio Cardarelli Hospital, Naples, Italy

AUTHORS

CLARE ARNOTT, MBBS(Hons), PhD
Associate Professor, Head of Heart Failure Program, The George Institute for Global Health, University of New South Wales, Newtown, Sydney, Australia; Department of Cardiology, Royal Prince Alfred Hospital, Sydney, Australia; Sydney Medical School, University of Sydney, New South Wales, Australia

CHRISTIAN-ALEXANDER BEHRENDT, MD, FESVS
Associate Professor, Head of Research Group GermanVasc, Department of Vascular Medicine, University Heart and Vascular Center UKE Hamburg, University Medical Center Hamburg-Eppendorf, Hamburg, Germany; Brandenburg Medical School Theodor Fontane, Neuruppin, Germany

AVIVIT CAHN, MD
The Faculty of Medicine, Hebrew University of Jerusalem, Diabetes Unit, Department of Endocrinology and Metabolism, Hadassah Medical Center, Jerusalem, Israel

FRANCESCO COSENTINO, MD, PhD
Professor, Division of Cardiology, Department of Medicine, Karolinska Institute, Heart, Vascular and Neuro Theme, Department of Cardiology, Karolinska University Hospital, Stockholm, Sweden

NEAL M. DIXIT, MD, MBA
Department of Medicine, David Geffen School of Medicine at UCLA, Los Angeles, California, USA

GIULIA FERRANNINI, MD
Division of Cardiology, Department of
Medicine, Karolinska Institute, Stockholm,
Sweden

ROBERT A. FLETCHER, MSc
Biostatistician, The George Institute for Global
Health, University of New South Wales,
Newtown, Sydney, Australia

GREGG C. FONAROW, MD
Department of Medicine, Division of
Cardiology, David Geffen School of Medicine
at UCLA, Los Angeles, California, USA

MARAT FUDIM, MD, MHS
Division of Cardiology, Department of
Medicine, Duke University, Duke Clinical
Research Institute, Durham, North Carolina,
USA

NICOLAS GIRERD, MD, PhD
Centre d'Investigation Clinique Pierre Drouin -
INSERM - CHRU de Nancy, Institut lorrain du
cœur et des vaisseaux Louis Mathieu, Nancy,
France

ALEXANDER GOMBERT, MD
European Vascular Centre Aachen-Maastricht,
Department of Vascular Surgery, University
Hospital RWTH Aachen, Aachen, Germany

JOSEPHINE L. HARRINGTON, MD
Duke Clinical Research Institute, Durham,
North Carolina, USA

NATALIA JARZEBSKA, M.Sc.
University Center for Vascular Medicine,
University Clinic Carl Gustav Carus,
Technische Universität Dresden, Germany

**PARDEEP S. JHUND, BSc, MBChB, MSc,
PhD**
BHF Cardiovascular Research Centre, Institute
of Cardiovascular and Medical Sciences,
University of Glasgow, Glasgow, United
Kingdom

AHMED A. KOLKAILAH, MD, MSc
The University of Texas Southwestern Medical
Center, Dallas, Texas, USA

CHIM C. LANG, MD
Professor of Cardiology, Head of Division,
Division of Molecular and Clinical Medicine,

School of Medicine, University of Dundee,
Dundee, United Kingdom

CHRISTINA MAGNUSSEN, MD
Department of Cardiology, University Heart
and Vascular Centre Hamburg, German Centre
for Cardiovascular Research (DZHK), Partner
Site Hamburg/Kiel/Luebeck, Hamburg,
Germany

ELENA MARCHIORI, MD
Department of Vascular and Endovascular
Surgery, University Hospital Münster, Münster,
Germany

DARREN K. McGUIRE, MD, MHSc
Professor, The University of Texas
Southwestern Medical Center, Parkland Health
and Hospital System, Dallas, Texas, USA

IFY R. MORDI, MD
Senior Lecturer in Cardiology, Division of
Molecular and Clinical Medicine, School of
Medicine, University of Dundee, Dundee,
United Kingdom

BRUCE NEAL, MB ChB, PhD
Professor, Executive Director, The George
Institute for Global Health, University of New
South Wales, Newtown, Sydney, Australia;
Department of Epidemiology and Biostatistics,
Imperial College London, London, United
Kingdom

ADAM J. NELSON, MBBS, MBA, MPH, PhD
Duke Clinical Research Institute, Durham,
North Carolina, USA

JOAKIM NORDANSTIG, MD, PhD
Institute of Medicine, Department of Molecular
and Clinical Medicine, University of
Gothenburg, Department of Vascular Surgery,
Sahlgrenska University Hospital, Gothenburg,
Sweden

NEHA J. PAGIDIPATI, MD, MPH
Duke Clinical Research Institute, Durham,
North Carolina, USA

FREDERIK PETERS, PhD
Research Group GermanVasc, Department of
Vascular Medicine, University Heart and
Vascular Center UKE Hamburg, University
Medical Center Hamburg-Eppendorf,
Hamburg, Germany

RENA POLLACK, MD
The Faculty of Medicine, Hebrew University
of Jerusalem, Department of Endocrinology
and Metabolism, Hadassah-Hebrew
University Medical Center, Jerusalem,
Israel

TRIPTI RASTOGI, MD, MSc
Centre d'Investigation Clinique Pierre Drouin -
INSERM - CHRU de Nancy, Institut lorrain du
cœur et des vaisseaux Louis Mathieu, Nancy,
France

ROMAN N. RODIONOV, MD, PhD, FAHA
University Center for Vascular Medicine,
University Clinic Carl Gustav Carus,
Technische Universität Dresden, Germany;
College of Medicine and Public Health, Flinders
University and Flinders Medical Centre,
Adelaide, Australia

HUSAM M. SALAH, MD
Department of Medicine, University of
Arkansas for Medical Sciences, Little Rock,
Arkansas, USA

GIANLUIGI SAVARESE, MD, PhD
Associate Professor, Division of Cardiology,
Department of Medicine, Karolinska Institute,
Heart, Vascular and Neuro Theme, Department
of Cardiology, Karolinska University Hospital,
Stockholm, Sweden

KONSTANTINOS SPANOS, MD, PhD
Vascular Surgery Department, Larissa
University Hospital, Faculty of Medicine,
School of Health Sciences, University of
Thessaly, Larissa, Greece

VOLKER VALLON, MD
Division of Nephrology and Hypertension,
Department of Medicine, Department of
Pharmacology, University of California, San
Diego, La Jolla, California, USA; VA San Diego
Healthcare System, San Diego, California, USA

BOBACK ZIAEIAN, MD, PhD
Department of Medicine, Division of Cardiology,
David Geffen School of Medicine at UCLA,
Division of Cardiology, VA Greater Los Angeles
Healthcare System, Los Angeles, California, USA

Contents

Sodium-glucose cotransporter 2 (SGLT2) inhibitors have consistently demonstrated improved outcomes in patients with heart failure with or without type 2 diabetes; however, the mechanisms contributing to these benefits remain poorly understood. Although SGLT2 inhibitors do have glucose-lowering effects, it is unlikely that their cardiovascular benefits are solely due to improved glycemic control. This improved glycemia leads to consequent metabolic effects that could provide further explanation for their action. This review discusses the glucose-lowering and metabolic effects of SGLT2 inhibitors and how these might lead to improved cardiovascular outcomes in patients with heart failure.

SGLT2 inhibitors can protect the kidneys of patients with and without type 2 diabetes from failing. This includes blood glucose dependent and independent mechanisms. SGLT2 inhibitors lower glomerular pressure and filtration, thereby reducing the physical stress on the filtration barrier and the oxygen demand for tubular reabsorption. This improves cortical oxygenation, which, together with lesser tubular glucotoxicity and improved mitochondrial function and autophagy, can reduce proinflammatory and profibrotic signaling and preserve tubular function and GFR in long term. By shifting transport downstream, SGLT2 inhibitors may mimic systemic hypoxia and stimulate erythropoiesis, which improves oxygen delivery to the kidney and other organs.

Sodium-glucose cotransporter 2 inhibitors were first discovered as glucose-lowering drugs because of their glycosuric action and good safety profile. Subsequently, they were studied in cardiovascular outcome trials in people with type 2 diabetes, and their cardiovascular benefit was consistently observed as regards heart failure hospitalizations and cardiovascular death. Investigation of the underlying mechanisms granting such benefit is continuously engaging researchers all over the world. The findings described in this article paved the way to a larger use of these drugs in patients with heart failure, with the aim of improving their clinical outcomes and quality of life.

Sodium-glucose transport inhibitors (SGLT2i) have been found to be effective in preventing heart failure in patients with diabetes or chronic kidney disease with or without cardiovascular disease. Recent evidence suggests that SGLT2i substantially improve cardiovascular and renal outcomes in patients with heart failure with reduced ejection fraction (HFrEF). In this review, we discuss the combined cardio-renal benefits of SGLT2i in patients with HFrEF. In addition, we discuss the impact of renoprotection in the midterm management of HFrEF and possible implementation strategies for initiating SGLT2i in routine care of HFrEF.

The trials of SLGT2 inhibitors in type 2 diabetes suggested a potential benefit of these drugs in patients with heart failure. When randomized trials confirmed their benefit in heart failure with reduced ejection fraction, attention turned to heart failure with preserved ejection fraction (HFPEF). In the EMPEROR-Preserved trial the SGLT2 inhibitor empagliflozin reduced the risk of cardiovascular death or hospitalization for heart failure (HR 0.79 95%CI 0.69–0.9, P < .001). This was driven by a reduction in worsening HF events. SGLT2 inhibitors are likely to become the new standard of care in patients with HFPEF.

Sodium-glucose cotransporter-2 inhibitors (SGLT2i) are a recent addition to the pillars of medical therapy for heart failure (HF) with reduced ejection fraction, all of which improve quality of life, morbidity, and mortality. These benefits are evident within the first 30 days of initiation. This review discusses the rationale for SGLT2i initiation in simultaneous or in rapid sequence with other guideline-directed medical therapy (GDMT). We also discuss SGLT2i use and early benefits in HF patients with an ejection fraction greater than 40%.

Sodium-glucose cotransporter-2 inhibitors (SGLT-2i) improve the risk for heart and kidney failure. However, their effects on major atherosclerotic cardiovascular events (MACE) are less clear. Although outcomes trials of drugs for diabetes were not powered to prove superiority, the totality of trial data yields an estimate of ~11% relative reduction for MACE (HR 0.89, 95%CI 0.82–0.96) and neutral on stroke (HR 0.92, 95%CI 0.79–1.08). In animal models, SGLT-2i favorably affects plaque size, composition, and inflammatory pathways; human data in this regard are lacking. Ongoing trials are evaluating SGLT-2i efficacy in heart failure, kidney disease, and postmyocardial infarction populations, independent of diabetes status.

Fifty articles comprising 18 randomized controlled trials (RCTs), 16 observational studies, and 16 meta-analyses on the safety and effectiveness of sodium-glucose cotransporter 2 inhibitors were evaluated in the current review. Only one-fourth of the cohorts of recent trials had peripheral arterial disease (PAD), whereas this subgroup was at high risk for amputations. Despite a remarkable heterogeneity of RCTs, only 2 trials on canagliflozin suggested excess amputation rates, whereas several observational studies generated conflicting conclusions and remained short on possible explanations. Preliminary evidence from observational research suggested that patients with PAD may even benefit from SGLT-2 inhibitor treatment due to lower observed heart failure hospitalization rates.

Nonalcoholic fatty liver disease (NAFLD) is a systemic disorder with cardiovascular manifestations; due to its complex and multifactorial pathophysiological mechanisms, no effective pharmacologic treatment has been identified to date. Sodium-glucose cotransporter 2 (SGLT2) inhibitors have demonstrated potentially favorable effects on NAFLD incidence and progression in preclinical and clinical studies. This review summarizes the evidence from preclinical and human studies supporting the use of SGLT2 inhibitors in NAFLD and proposes several mechanisms that may drive these favorable effects (ie, increasing insulin sensitivity, decreasing intrahepatic fat accumulation and lipotoxicity, decreasing oxidative stress and endoplasmic reticulum (ER) stress, improving autophagy, and inhibiting apoptosis).

SGLT2 inhibitors (SGLT2i) are effective in the management of diabetes and in reducing adverse cardiovascular and renal outcomes. Randomized clinical trials demonstrated safety and tolerability in older adults. Adverse effects associated with SGLT2i are impacted by patient frailty, comorbidities, and concomitant medication use and, therefore, must be thoroughly evaluated before initiating treatment. The risk of volume depletion, hypoglycemia, genital infections, and diabetic ketoacidosis can be minimized by appropriate patient selection, patient education, and early symptom recognition. Limited data exists regarding the risk of urinary tract infections, fractures, and amputations in the elderly treated with SGLT2i and routine monitoring is recommended.

Sodium glucose cotransporter 2 (SGLT2) inhibitors are associated with cardiovascular and renal benefits across a broad range of patients, with no increase in total serious adverse events. We evaluated the evidence with respect to amputation and fracture risks for this drug class. Overall, SGLT2 inhibitors are not associated with an increased risk of amputation or fracture in any of the patient populations they have been tested in. The increase in amputation and fracture risks with canagliflozin observed in the CANagliflozin cardioVascular Assessment Study (CANVAS) program was not seen in the Canagliflozin and Renal Events in Diabetes with Established Nephropathy Clinical Evaluation trial or any study of other SGLT2 inhibitors. Extensive evaluation of amputation and fracture risks suggests that the CANVAS program findings were chance observations rather than real effects.

HEART FAILURE CLINICS

Preface
SGLT2 Inhibitors Are Lifesavers in Heart Failure

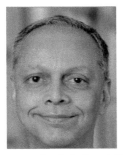
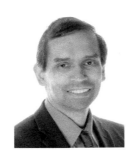
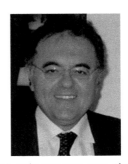

Ragavendra R. Baliga, MD, MBA, FACP, FRCP (Edin), FACC

Deepak L. Bhatt, MD, MPH, FACC, FAHA, FSCAI, FESC

Eduardo Bossone, MD, PhD, FCCP, FESC, FACC

Editors

The first three trials of sodium-glucose cotransporter-2 (SGLT2) inhibitors investigating cardiovascular (CV) safety, as required by the Food and Drug Administration, all revealed an unexpected approximate 30% reduction in heart failure (HF) hospitalizations in patients with type 2 diabetes mellitus (T2DM) with and at risk for CV disease.[1–3] However, these drugs were not associated with decreased stroke risk or reductions in myocardial infarction. These findings piqued the interest of HF specialists and led to clinical trials specifically investigating the effects of SGLT2 inhibitors in patients with HF (**Fig. 1**).[4–10]

In the DAPA-HF trial reported in the *New England Journal of Medicine* in November 2019,[4] the investigators found that in patients with *symptomatic* heart failure with reduced ejection fraction (HFrEF), dapagliflozin was beneficial in that dapagliflozin versus placebo was associated with a reduction in CV deaths and HF events, recurrent HF events, and ventricular arrhythmias, and also was associated with improvement in symptoms. These benefits were consistent across the age spectrum, risk spectrum, baseline diuretic use, baseline use of sacubitril/valsartan (although only 10% of the study cohort was on this combination), and mineralocorticoid receptor antagonists (MRAs). There was no sign of excess adverse safety events with these combinations of drugs. A subgroup analysis indicated that the benefit seen was independent of the presence or absence of diabetes. Almost all the patients had moderate

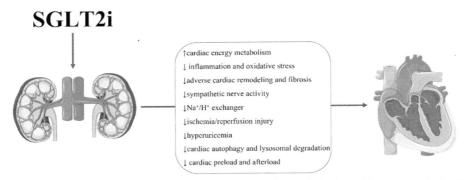

Fig. 1. Myocardial direct and indirect effects of SGLT2 inhibitors (SGLT2i). (*Adapted from* Lopaschuk GD, Verma S. Mechanisms of Cardiovascular Benefits of Sodium Glucose Co-Transporter 2 (SGLT2) Inhibitors: A State-of-the-Art Review. JACC Basic Transl Sci. 2020 Jun 22;5(6):632-644.)

Heart Failure Clin 18 (2022) xi–xiv
https://doi.org/10.1016/j.hfc.2022.07.001
1551-7136/22/© 2022 Published by Elsevier Inc.

HF, so the benefit and side-effect profile in patients with more severe HF was not studied.

The results of EMPEROR-REDUCED trial[7] indicated that empagliflozin was superior to placebo in improving HF outcomes among patients with symptomatic stable HFrEF (EF $\leq$ 40%) on excellent baseline guideline-directed medical therapy, irrespective of diabetes status. Benefit was primarily driven by a reduction in HF hospitalizations, not mortality. There was an early and sustained benefit on KCCQ-CSS. There was also a benefit in kidney outcomes. The use of MRAs did not influence the effect of empagliflozin on clinical outcomes. Even patients with severe left ventricular dysfunction appeared to benefit; the trial enrolled patients with an average ejection fraction (EF) of 27%, and greater than 70% of patients had an EF $\leq$30%; patients with EF greater than 30% were only included if they had an HF hospitalization in the prior 12 months and met specific natriuretic peptide benchmarks. A higher rate of genital mycotic infections was observed with SGLT2 inhibition, as had been previously reported with multiple other trials in this class.

Of note, the DAPA-HF trial was larger and did show a benefit in CV and all-cause mortality with dapagliflozin use. The subgroup analysis of the EMPEROR-REDUCED trial suggested that this benefit may not necessarily be driven by a diuretic effect alone (as noted among patients with and without recent volume overload), but further studies are needed to clarify this and other potential mechanisms of benefit. The cardiorenal benefits could be due to a combination of several factors, including a decrease in arterial stiffness, increase in hematocrit, decreased glucotoxicity, increase in weight loss, decrease in inflammation, increase in circulating provascular progenitor cells,[11] and decrease in circulating plasma volume with lower potential for developing volume depletion.[12]

SOLOIST-WHF was the first large, randomized controlled trial to show that initiation of SGLT2 inhibition in *acute HF* in stabilized patients prior to discharge or shortly thereafter is safe and effective. The benefits were consistent in those with not only HFrEF but also heart failure with preserved ejection fraction (HFpEF). Sotagliflozin is an SGLT2 inhibitor, but also inhibits SGLT1, which is expressed in the gut and delays glucose absorption. The goal of the trial was to assess the safety and efficacy of sotagliflozin in reducing CV events among patients with T2DM and recent HF admission. The primary endpoint of total CV death, hospitalization for HF, or urgent visit for HF for sotagliflozin versus placebo was 70 versus 98 events/100 patient-years (hazard ratio, 0.67; 95% confidence interval, 0.52–0.85; P = .0009). This achieved significance by *28 days of follow-up*. There was also a significant improvement in the KCCQ[9] and in days alive and outside of the hospital.[13] In the pooled analysis of SCORED and SOLOIST-WHF data, benefits were present irrespective of baseline EF (including among patients with HFpEF) and prior history of HF. Empagliflozin has also been found to be beneficial in acute HF.[14]

The Framingham study reported that 10% of the patients with HF die within the first month and 20% to 30% die within the first year.[15] Similar findings have been reported recently,[16] and 1 in 4 US patients hospitalized for HF die or are rehospitalized within 30 days of discharge,[17] making it important that the therapy of acute HF be urgent. Given that mortality in acute HF is high in the first month after diagnosis, the early benefit of SGLT2 inhibitors in HF makes it important that therapy is started early. In DAPA-HF, there was a 49% reduction in events (worsening HF or CV death) by day 28. In the EMPEROR-Reduced trial, the benefit of reduction in combined risk of death, hospitalization for HF, or an emergent/urgent HF visit reached statistical significance at 12 days after randomization. In SOLOIST-WHF, there was a 39% reduction in events (total CV death, HHF, and urgent HF visit) by 28 days. These studies have prompted the call for early initiation of SGLT2 inhibitor therapy in HF.[18–21]

The pooled analysis of EMPEROR-Reduced and EMPEROR-Preserved suggests that the kidney benefit is primarily among patients with HFrEF,[5] and eGFR slope analysis may not be predictive of kidney outcomes among patients with HF. The SCORED trial showed that sotagliflozin has beneficial effects on CV outcomes among patients with T2DM and chronic kidney disease. The benefit was primarily in reduction of HF events, but there was also a reduction in CV death/myocardial infarction/stroke, primarily owing to reduction in MI and stroke. A reduction in kidney events was not observed, likely owing to early cessation of the trial because of loss of funding. The significant reduction in kidney disease progression has also been shown in CREDENCE[22] and DAPA-CKD,[23] indicating an expanded role for SGLT2 is in nephrology practice as adjunctive agents to slow the progression of kidney disease.

To discuss these salutary benefits of SGLT2 inhibitors in detail, we have assembled a terrific panel of international experts on this new class of therapeutic agents. We hope these articles will persuade you all to consider, in appropriate patients, early initiation of these lifesavers.

Ragavendra R. Baliga, MD, MBA, FACP, FRCP
(Edin), FACC
Division of Cardiology
The Ohio State University
Wexner Medical Center
Columbus, OH, USA

Deepak L. Bhatt, MD, MPH, FACC, FAHA, FSCAI,
FESC
Brigham and Women's Hospital Heart &
Vascular Center
Harvard Medical School
75 Francis Street
Boston, MA, USA

Eduardo Bossone, MD, PhD, FCCP, FESC, FACC
Cardarelli Hospital
Naples, Italy

E-mail addresses:
rrbaliga@gmail.com (R.R. Baliga)
dlbhattmd@post.harvard.edu (D.L. Bhatt)
ebossone@hotmail.com (E. Bossone)

REFERENCES

1. Zinman B, Wanner C, Lachin JM, et al. Empagliflozin, cardiovascular outcomes, and mortality in type 2 diabetes. N Engl J Med 2015;373(22):2117–28. https://doi.org/10.1056/NEJMoa1504720 Epub 20150917. PubMed PMID: 26378978.

2. Neal B, Perkovic V, Mahaffey KW, et al. Canagliflozin and cardiovascular and renal events in type 2 diabetes. N Engl J Med 2017;377(7):644–57. https://doi.org/10.1056/NEJMoa1611925 Epub 20170612. PubMed PMID: 28605608.

3. Wiviott SD, Raz I, Bonaca MP, et al. Dapagliflozin and cardiovascular outcomes in type 2 diabetes. N Engl J Med 2019;380(4):347–57. https://doi.org/10.1056/NEJMoa1812389 Epub 20181110. PubMed PMID: 30415602.

4. McMurray JJV, Solomon SD, Inzucchi SE, et al. Dapagliflozin in patients with heart failure and reduced ejection fraction. N Engl J Med 2019;381(21):1995–2008. https://doi.org/10.1056/NEJMoa1911303 Epub 20190919. PubMed PMID: 31535829.

5. Zannad F, Ferreira JP, Pocock SJ, et al. SGLT2 inhibitors in patients with heart failure with reduced ejection fraction: a meta-analysis of the EMPEROR-reduced and DAPA-HF trials. Lancet 2020;396(10254):819–29. https://doi.org/10.1016/S0140-6736(20)31824-9 Epub 20200830. PubMed PMID: 32877652.

6. Packer M, Butler J, Zannad F, et al. Empagliflozin and major renal outcomes in heart failure. N Engl J Med 2021;385(16):1531–3. https://doi.org/10.1056/NEJMc2112411 Epub 20210827. PubMed PMID: 34449179.

7. Packer M, Anker SD, Butler J, et al. Cardiovascular and renal outcomes with empagliflozin in heart failure. N Engl J Med 2020;383(15):1413–24. https://doi.org/10.1056/NEJMoa2022190 Epub 20200828. PubMed PMID: 32865377.

8. Anker SD, Butler J, Filippatos G, et al. Empagliflozin in heart failure with a preserved ejection fraction. N Engl J Med 2021;385(16):1451–61. https://doi.org/10.1056/NEJMoa2107038 Epub 20210827. PubMed PMID: 34449189.

9. Bhatt DL, Szarek M, Steg PG, et al. Sotagliflozin in patients with diabetes and recent worsening heart failure. N Engl J Med 2021;384(2):117–28. https://doi.org/10.1056/NEJMoa2030183 Epub 20201116. PubMed PMID: 33200892.

10. Bhatt DL, Szarek M, Pitt B, et al. Sotagliflozin in patients with diabetes and chronic kidney disease. N Engl J Med 2021;384(2):129–39. https://doi.org/10.1056/NEJMoa2030186 Epub 20201116. PubMed PMID: 33200891.

11. Hess DA, Terenzi DC, Trac JZ, et al. SGLT2 inhibition with empagliflozin increases circulating provascular progenitor cells in people with type 2 diabetes mellitus. Cell Metab 2019;30(4):609–13. https://doi.org/10.1016/j.cmet.2019.08.015 Epub 20190830. PubMed PMID: 31477497.

12. Zelniker TA, Braunwald E. Mechanisms of cardiorenal effects of sodium-glucose cotransporter 2 inhibitors: JACC state-of-the-art review. J Am Coll Cardiol 2020;75(4):422–34. https://doi.org/10.1016/j.jacc.2019.11.031 PubMed PMID: 32000955.

13. Szarek M, Bhatt DL, Steg PG, et al. Effect of sotagliflozin on total hospitalizations in patients with type 2 diabetes and worsening heart failure: a randomized trial. Ann Intern Med 2021;174(8):1065–72. https://doi.org/10.7326/M21-0651 Epub 20210622. PubMed PMID: 34152828.

14. Voors AA, Angermann CE, Teerlink JR, et al. The SGLT2 inhibitor empagliflozin in patients hospitalized for acute heart failure: a multinational randomized trial. Nat Med 2022. https://doi.org/10.1038/s41591-021-01659-1. Epub 20220228. PubMed PMID: 35228754.

15. Levy D, Kenchaiah S, Larson MG, et al. Long-term trends in the incidence of and survival with heart failure. N Engl J Med 2002;347(18):1397–402. https://doi.org/10.1056/NEJMoa020265 PubMed PMID: 12409541.

16. Conrad N, Judge A, Canoy D, et al. Temporal trends and patterns in mortality after incident heart failure: a longitudinal analysis of 86 000 individuals. JAMA Cardiol 2019;4(11):1102–11. https://doi.org/10.1001/jamacardio.2019.3593 PubMed PMID: 31479100; PubMed Central PMCID: PMC6724155.

17. Wadhera RK, Joynt Maddox KE, Wasfy JH, et al. Association of the hospital readmissions reduction program with mortality among Medicare beneficiaries hospitalized for heart failure, acute myocardial infarction, and pneumonia. JAMA 2018;320(24): 2542–52. https://doi.org/10.1001/jama.2018.19232 PubMed PMID: 30575880; PubMed Central PMCID: PMC6583517.

18. McMurray JJV, Packer M. How should we sequence the treatments for heart failure and a reduced ejection fraction?: A redefinition of evidence-based medicine. Circulation 2021;143(9):875–7. https://doi.org/10.1161/CIRCULATIONAHA.120.052926 Epub 20201230. PubMed PMID: 33378214.

19. Greene SJ, Butler J, Fonarow GC. Simultaneous or rapid sequence initiation of quadruple medical therapy for heart failure-optimizing therapy with the need for speed. JAMA Cardiol 2021;6(7):743–4. https://doi.org/10.1001/jamacardio.2021.0496 PubMed PMID: 33787823.

20. Baliga R. Door-to-GDMT time & door to max-dose GDMT time. Available at: https://youtu.be/HM-bdHScVdE. In: RR B, editor. Dr RR Baliga's 'GOT KNOWLEDGE DOC" Podkast. YouTube: MasterMed-facts.com; 2021. Accessed.

21. Verma S, Anker SD, Butler J, et al. Early initiation of SGLT2 inhibitors is important, irrespective of ejection fraction: SOLOIST-WHF in perspective. ESC Heart Failure 2020;7(6):3261–7. https://doi.org/10.1002/ehf2.13148 PubMed PMID: PMC7754955.

22. Perkovic V, Jardine MJ, Neal B, et al. Canagliflozin and renal outcomes in type 2 diabetes and nephropathy. N Engl J Med 2019;380(24):2295–306. https://doi.org/10.1056/NEJMoa1811744 Epub 20190414. PubMed PMID: 30990260.

23. Heerspink HJL, Stefánsson BV, Correa-Rotter R, et al. Dapagliflozin in patients with chronic kidney disease. N Engl J Med 2020;383(15):1436–46. https://doi.org/10.1056/NEJMoa2024816 Epub 20200924. PubMed PMID: 32970396.

Glucose-Lowering and Metabolic Effects of SGLT2 Inhibitors

Ify R. Mordi, MD, Chim C. Lang, MD*

KEYWORDS

- SGLT2 inhibitors • Glycemia • Cardiometabolic • Heart failure

KEY POINTS

- SGLT2 inhibitors have consistently been shown to improve cardiovascular outcomes in patients with heart failure with and without diabetes.
- The cardiovascular benefits seem to be driven by factors beyond simple glucose lowering or changes in conventional cardiovascular risk factors.
- The glucose-lowering effects of SGLT2 inhibitors cause several potentially beneficial systemic and cardiac metabolic changes that could in part help explain the cardiac benefits of SGLT2 inhibitors.

INTRODUCTION

Sodium-glucose cotransporter 2 (SGLT2) inhibitors were initially developed as a glucose-lowering diabetes therapy. Subsequent cardiovascular (CV) outcome trials demonstrated a striking, consistent beneficial CV risk reduction, in particular a reduction in heart failure (HF) hospitalization. These benefits have been confirmed in patients with HF with both reduced and preserved ejection fraction with and without diabetes.[1–3]

The consistent results from these clinical trials suggest that there is likely a class effect from SGLT2 inhibitors. How SGLT2 inhibitors exert their remarkable benefits on CV outcome is still poorly understood. For example, only 12% of the relative risk reduction for all-cause death can be explained by the combined changes in conventional CV risk factors.[4] The benefits in patients without diabetes suggest that the mechanisms by which SGLT2 inhibitors exert their beneficial effects are likely beyond simple glucose lowering. Although many potential mechanisms for these effects have been postulated, the exact pathways by which SGLT2 inhibitors improve CV outcome remain unclear. Outcome trial data in patients with HF suggest several potentially beneficial contributing effects, summarized in **Table 1**; however, as described earlier, these changes may only account for a modest contribution. The primary action of SGLT2 inhibitors on glucose reabsorption that causes their glucose-lowering effects also has several metabolic consequences that may help further explain their CV benefits. The aim of this review is to discuss both the glucose-lowering and metabolic effects of SGLT2 inhibitors, focusing predominantly on clinical data.

GLUCOSE-LOWERING EFFECTS

The association between diabetes, dysglycemia, and development of HF is well established. As well as its associated comorbidities such as coronary artery disease, diabetes and dysglycemia themselves are associated with myocardial changes (sometimes termed *diabetic cardiomyopathy*).[5] Although the pathophysiology of diabetic cardiomyopathy is itself not completely

Dr I.R. Mordi has received speaker fees from Boehringer Ingelheim, United Kingdom and research funding from Astra Zeneca, United Kingdom. Dr C.C. Lang has received consultancy and speaker fees and research funding from AstraZeneca, Boehringer Ingelheim, and Novo Nordisk, Denmark and consultancy and speaker fees from MSD, United Kingdom.
Division of Molecular and Clinical Medicine, School of Medicine, University of Dundee, Dundee DD1 9SY, United Kingdom
* Corresponding author.
E-mail address: c.c.lang@dundee.ac.uk

Heart Failure Clin 18 (2022) 529–538
https://doi.org/10.1016/j.hfc.2022.03.004

Table 1
Summary of changes in glycemic and metabolic parameters versus placebo in SGLT2 heart failure outcome trials

	DAPA-HF[3]	EMPEROR-Reduced[2]	EMPEROR-Preserved[1]
	Dapagliflozin	Empagliflozin	Empagliflozin
Median duration of follow-up	18 mo	16 mo	26 mo
HbA$_{1c}$ (%) in patients with T2D	−0.24 (−0.34 to −0.13)	−0.16 (−0.25 to −0.08)	−0.19 (−0.25 to −0.14)
Hypoglycemia (active/placebo) %	0.2/0.2	1.4/1.5 (T2D) 0.7/0.6 (No T2D)	4.3/4.5 (T2D) 0.7/0.8 (No T2D)
New-onset diabetes (active/placebo) %	4.9/7.1 (All patients)	11.2/12.6 (Prediabetes only)	12.0/14.0 (Prediabetes only)
Body weight (kg)	−0.87 (−1.11 to −0.62)	−0.82 (−1.18 to −0.45)	−1.28 (−1.54 to −1.03)
Systolic blood pressure (mm Hg)	−0.87 (−1.11 to −0.62)	−0.7 (−1.8–0.4)	−1.2 (−2.1 to −0.3)
Hematocrit (%)	2.41 (2.21–2.62)	2.36 (2.08–2.63)	2.36 (2.17–2.54)

Abbreviations: HbA$_{1c}$, glycated hemoglobin; T2D, type 2 diabetes.

understood, postulated mechanisms include coronary artery disease, advanced glycation end products, microvascular function, lipotoxicity, fibrosis, altered myocardial metabolism, insulin resistance, oxidative stress, and inflammation that lead to adverse remodeling and diastolic and systolic dysfunction.[6]

Clearly, because they were initially designed as type 2 diabetes (T2D) medications, the obvious initial mechanistic explanation for the beneficial effects of SGLT2 inhibitors might be their effects on glycemic control. If this solely were the case, however, one might expect that other glucose-lowering drugs might also be beneficial in HF, and this is not the case. The primary action of SGLT2 inhibitors is in the proximal convoluted tubule, causing increased glycosuria and decreased serum glucose. Theoretically, increased glycosuria might reduce cardiac glucotoxicity, reducing vascular dysfunction and oxidative stress.[7] Nevertheless, the reduction in glycated hemoglobin (HbA$_{1c}$) with SGLT2 inhibitors is modest compared with other classes such as glucagonlike peptide-1 agonists.[8] In the major CV outcome trials, SGLT2 inhibitors reduced HbA$_{1c}$ by around 0.5%. As would be expected, the consistent improvement in glycemic control seen in the diabetes CV outcome trials was replicated in patients with diabetes in the HF trials. In patients with T2D in DAPA-HF, dapagliflozin caused a 0.24% reduction in HbA1c, whereas in EMPEROR-Reduced the reduction with empagliflozin was 0.16%. Although these reductions were more than in the placebo groups, the early benefit seen with SGLT2 inhibitors in these HF trials (within 3 months), in conjunction with the overall improvement in outcomes in patients with HF without diabetes, suggests that improvements in glycemic control are unlikely to be the major mechanism underlying the positive trial results.

Data from large outcome trials in patients with HF suggest that SGLT2 inhibitors may also prevent new-onset diabetes in patients with HF without T2D at baseline. Given the increased mortality associated with diabetes and its complications in patients with HF,[9,10] preventing diabetes development could further improve long-term CV outcome. In the subset of patients without diabetes in DAPA-HF, dapagliflozin caused a 32% reduction in incident diabetes versus placebo.[11] Most patients who developed diabetes had prediabetes at baseline (defined as HbA$_{1c}$ 5.7%–6.4%), and development of diabetes was associated with increased mortality. In addition, dapagliflozin did not cause a significant change in HbA$_{1c}$ in this group (−0.04%), suggesting that improved glycemic control is unlikely to be relevant in patients with HF without diabetes. There was also numerically lower incidence of new-onset diabetes in patients with prediabetes randomized to empagliflozin versus placebo in both EMPEROR-Reduced[2] and EMPEROR-Preserved.[1]

Overall, although SGLT2 inhibitors do provide a favorable glycemic profile, the likelihood is that the mechanisms explaining their CV benefit lie beyond simple glucose lowering.

METABOLIC EFFECTS

The glycosuric effect of SGLT2 inhibitors resulting in a mild caloric restriction leads to several additional adaptive responses that have effects on metabolism.[12] By reducing overall glucotoxicity SGLT2 inhibition may improve insulin sensitivity by increasing insulin secretion and improving pancreatic beta cell function.[13] The changes seem to be predominantly mediated by the overall reduction in plasma glucose rather than any direct effects on the pancreas.[14] These favorable changes also lead to improvements in hepatic[15] and peripheral muscle insulin sensitivity[16] and a shift from glucose to lipid oxidation and a consequent increase in plasma ketones.[17] These metabolic changes provide the basis for some mechanistic insight as to the potential mechanisms of benefit in patients with HF. These metabolic effects can be divided into cardiac effects and systemic effects.

CARDIAC METABOLIC EFFECTS
Myocardial Energetics

In healthy conditions, most myocardial metabolism uses free fatty acids and glucose; however, in T2D and HF fatty acid and glucose uptake and oxidation is impaired.[18] In this setting, ketone bodies become a more efficient myocardial energy substrate. Serum levels of ketone bodies increase in patients with diabetes after SGLT2 inhibitor treatment, due to a reduction in hepatic ketone synthesis and decreased ketonuria.[19] One hypothesized mechanism for the benefits of SGLT2 inhibitors in HF is that increased ketosis shifts myocardial metabolism toward preferential use of ketones such as beta-hydroxybutyrate.[20] Increased ketosis has been confirmed in patients with HF in the REFORM trial, in which dapagliflozin caused an increase in beta-hydroxybutyrate.[21] A more recent study designed to explore this hypothesis further in a cohort of stable patients with HF, however, reported that although empagliflozin caused an increase in beta-hydroxybutyrate, this actually attenuated the empagliflozin-derived decreases in systolic blood pressure (SBP) compared with placebo.[22]

A recent study in patients with T2D used CV MRI to evaluate the myocardial metabolic effects of empagliflozin.[23] In this observational study the investigators found that 12 weeks of empagliflozin therapy was associated with improvement in myocardial energetics (measured by phosphocreatinine to adenosine triphosphate ratio), as well as significant improvements in left ventricular volumes and global longitudinal strain. The mean left ventricular ejection fraction in this cohort was 52%. There was no difference in myocardial blood flow, suggesting that these metabolic changes

were not due to improvements in microvascular perfusion.

Although these data certainly hint that SGLT2 inhibitors may have direct myocardial metabolic effects, as yet there have not been any large studies in patients with HF. The upcoming EMPA-VISION trial (NCT03332212) will report on the effects of empagliflozin on various metabolic parameters in both heart failure with reduced ejection fraction (HFrEF) and heart failure with preserved ejection fraction (HFpEF) patients, with a primary outcome of change in resting phosphocreatine-to-adenosine triphosphate ratio, as measured by 31-phosphorus magnetic resonance spectroscopy.[24] This study will shed light on whether some of the beneficial CV effects of SGLT2 inhibitors may be caused by direct improvements in myocardial metabolism. Changes in intracellular calcium homeostasis have also been implicated in HF.[25] Another study (NCT04591639) will assess whether beneficial changes in calcium handling might also occur with dapagliflozin.

Inflammation, Oxidative Stress, and Fibrosis

Systemic inflammation and oxidative stress are important in the pathophysiology of HF, leading to myocardial tissue damage, fibrosis, adverse remodeling, and eventually left ventricular dysfunction.[26–29] SGLT2 inhibitors seem to also have systemic anti-inflammatory effects that might explain some of the benefit.

Kolijn and colleagues[30] reported in a study using a murine model of HFpEF and in human myocardial tissue that empagliflozin reduced inflammation and oxidative stress (via the nitric oxide, sodium guanylate cyclase, and cyclic GMP pathways), and consequently reduced myocardial stiffness. In a randomized clinical trial empagliflozin reduced high-sensitivity C-reactive protein (hsCRP) levels by 54% at 12 months compared with placebo in individuals with T2D at high CV risk, as well as reduced insulin resistance measured by the homeostatic model assessment of insulin resistance (HOMA-IR).[31] These changes were also associated with improvements in SBP and high-density lipoprotein cholesterol levels (although there was no change in low-density lipoprotein cholesterol levels). Similar results were reported in the DAPA-LVH trial, in which compared with placebo, dapagliflozin caused significant reductions in hsCRP and HOMA-IR in a cohort of patients with T2D and left ventricular hypertrophy.[32]

As well as reducing inflammation, SGLT2 inhibitors may have beneficial effects on peripheral vasculature. Empagliflozin also caused improvements in aortic stiffness (reduced pulse wave velocity) in EMPA-TROPISM.[33] In a non-randomized case-control study SGLT2 inhibitors were associated with significant improvements in endothelial function measured by flow-mediated dilation.[34] Other studies have reported conflicting results, however, including randomized trials.[35] Empagliflozin did not cause a significant change in endothelial function measured by reactive hyperemia index after 24 weeks in a randomized trial of diabetic patients with established CV disease.[36] A recent analysis of the EMPA-HEART Cardiolink-6 trial provided evidence suggesting that one possible mechanism of benefit might be reversal of regenerative cell exhaustion caused by oxidative stress in the endothelium.[37] Further work is required to identify whether changes in endothelial function or arterial stiffness play a role in HF.

SYSTEMIC EFFECTS
Weight Loss

Obesity and adiposity are established as risk factors for incident HF (in particular HFpEF), causing left ventricular structural and functional abnormalities predisposing to HF.[38,39] Despite this, the "obesity paradox" has been reported in numerous observational studies suggesting that the lower body mass index is associated with increased mortality in patients with HF.[40] Obesity drives HF development via the frequent presence of concomitant risk factors such as diabetes, coronary artery disease, and hypertension, and also by direct changes in the myocardium. These changes include cardiomyocyte hypertrophy, fibrosis, and inflammation.[41] The location and distribution of fat also plays a role in the HF pathophysiology. Epicardial adipose is increasingly recognized as an important risk factor for CV disease, possibly related to increased arterial stiffness and inflammation, and is associated with adverse prognosis in patients with HF.[42,43] Visceral adipose tissue is also more strongly associated with incident HF than subcutaneous adipose.[44,45]

In diabetic patients SGLT2 inhibitors consistently cause weight loss, predominantly caused by body fat loss.[46] Meta-analyses suggest that the expected weight loss is around 2 kg versus placebo, and that this weight loss is sustained up to 4 years.[47,48] This weight loss was also seen in the CV outcome trials, alongside a reduction in waist/hip ratio. Beyond a simple reduction in body weight, SGLT2 inhibitors may also affect body fat composition including reducing visceral adipose.[49] In an ex vivo study dapagliflozin was found to increase epicardial

adipose glucose uptake and reduce secretion of proinflammatory cytokines.[50] SGLT2 inhibitors may also cause favorable changes within adipose vasculature.[51]

In patients with HF, the benefits of SGLT2 inhibitors seem to be consistent regardless of the body mass index (BMI). In DAPA-HF dapagliflozin caused a mean weight loss of 0.9 kg versus placebo, which was independent of baseline BMI.[52] There was also no significant difference in the effect of dapagliflozin on SBP, hematocrit, or heart rate based on baseline BMI. Similar reductions in body weight were seen in EMPEROR-Reduced and EMPEROR-Preserved (0.8 and 1.3 kg, respectively), and again, there was no significant interaction of the effect of empagliflozin on the primary outcome. Beyond overall weight reduction, in a secondary analysis of the EMPA-TROPISM trial empagliflozin was associated with significant reductions in epicardial and subcutaneous adipose compared with placebo, as well as with reductions in extracellular matrix and cardiomyocyte volume, in patients with HFrEF without diabetes.[33]

Overall, although weight loss is probably beneficial in this setting, given the modest effects on weight from SGLT2 inhibitors and the consistent outcome benefit regardless of baseline weight, it is unlikely that this explains the whole mechanism of benefit. Changes in epicardial adipose and body fat distribution may well be a contributor.

Liver/Metabolic Syndrome

T2D is associated with metabolic syndrome, a key component of which is insulin resistance, which is related to myocardial structural and functional changes that lead to HF.[53,54] Insulin resistance is an important driver of HF, with a study of 550 individuals finding that normal-weight individuals with insulin resistance had a higher risk of incident HF than overweight or obese individuals without metabolic syndrome.[55] SGLT2 inhibitors seem to improve pancreatic beta cell function, potentially reducing insulin resistance and protecting against further dysfunction.[13,56] In EMPA-REG the effect of empagliflozin was consistent regardless of the presence of metabolic syndrome (82% of participants had metabolic syndrome).[57] By improving insulin sensitivity overall, SGLT2 inhibitors may provide benefit. SGLT2 inhibitors increase endogenous glucose production and reduce systemic glucotoxicity, providing further systemic metabolic benefits.[58]

SGLT2 inhibitors may also reduce hepatic fat, a particularly relevant contributor to disease. In patients with T2D dapagliflozin cause significant reductions in liver biomarkers and hepatic fat, as well as improves peripheral insulin sensitivity.[59–61] Nonalcoholic fatty liver disease has a bidirectional relationship with HF, and therefore this mechanism may also play an important role.[62]

Diuresis/Hemoconcentration

By blocking glucose reabsorption in the proximal convoluted tubule SGLT2 inhibitors cause an osmotic diuresis, in particular glucosuria, leading to their glycemic effects.[63] This diuretic effect could clearly be beneficial in HF, and might explain the early benefit seen in HF outcome trials, due to improvement in ventricular loading conditions. This diuresis is additional to loop diuretics, which are commonly prescribed in patients with HF. We demonstrated, in the RECEDE-CHF trial including patients with HF and T2D, that by day 3 empagliflozin caused a significant increase in 24-hour urine volume compared with placebo (535 mL) and that this persisted to week 6, hinting at a potential reason for the early improvement in outcome seen in the large trials.[64] This increase was not accompanied by an increase in natriuresis, a finding replicated in other studies, suggesting that glycosuria is indeed the main mechanism of diuresis rather than natriuresis.[65,66] SGLT2 inhibitors may also offer a particularly favorable diuretic profile. Mathematical modeling studies have suggested that they preferentially reduce interstitial fluid (rather than causing intravascular depletion), which might be of added benefit in HF.[67] Supporting this, in RECEDE-CHF we found that empagliflozin caused a significant increase in electrolyte-free water clearance after 6 weeks.[64] In a small study by Jensen and colleagues[68] empagliflozin reduced estimated extracellular volume after 12 weeks compared with placebo.

Diuresis and hemoconcentration may also have other benefits. In DAPA-LVH, dapagliflozin caused a significant improvement in left ventricular systolic function (measured by global longitudinal strain) compared with placebo, and this correlated with an increase in hematocrit.[69] In EMPEROR-Reduced empagliflozin increased both hematocrit and hemoglobin compared with placebo early in the trial and prevented new-onset anemia.[70] The increase in hematocrit was, however, not associated with changes in body weight, N-Terminal Pro B-type Natriuretic Peptide (NT-proBNP), or blood pressure, and so it was postulated that the hematocrit increase is not simply due to hemoconcentration but may be explained by other mechanisms such as reduced renal oxidative stress and stimulation of erythropoiesis.[71]

In summary, although SGLT2 inhibitors certainly have a favorable diuretic effect that one would expect to contribute to initial benefit, their benefits seem to be independent of background diuretic therapy. Furthermore, the diuretic effect may not explain the longer-term benefits seen in the large outcome trials.

Blood Pressure

Hypertension and is strongly implicated as a risk factor for both HFrEF and HFpEF.[72] Chronically high SBP leads to an increase in afterload, left ventricular hypertrophy, and diastolic dysfunction that all predispose to incident HF. In patients with HF, the relationship is less clear, with numerous population studies identifying a J-shaped relationship between SBP and outcomes, with both high and low SBP being associated with adverse events in patients with HF.[73] Hypertension is more common in HFpEF, and it may be that lower SBP (particularly in HFrEF) is simply a reflection of a lower cardiac output and a marker of the patient being more unwell. Hypotension is more prevalent in patients with HFrEF and indeed can often limit the use of other HF therapies, therefore the favorable effect profile of SGLT2 inhibitors on SBP is a particular strength of this drug class.

Over the duration of EMPEROR-Reduced empagliflozin caused a small reduction in SBP, although across the whole study population this was not significantly different from placebo (−2.4 mm Hg vs −1.7 mm Hg, respectively). Further analysis of SBP response found that SBP actually increased in patients with SBP less than 110 mm Hg at baseline and decreased in those with SBP greater than 130 mm Hg at baseline.[74] Empagliflozin was not associated with an increase in symptomatic hypotension, underscoring its favorable blood pressure profile. Dapagliflozin seemed to have a slightly stronger effect on SBP, with a mean difference of −1.4 mm Hg at 8 months across all patients in DAPA-HF, which was significantly different to placebo, and again the magnitude of SBP reduction was larger in those with baseline SBP greater than 130 mm Hg.[75] The SBP reduction caused by empagliflozin was similar to that caused by dapagliflozin, whereas the there was a larger SBP reduction in the placebo group in EMPEROR-Reduced, which might explain the slight differences in results. Importantly, the CV and renal benefits seen with SGLT2 inhibitors in patients with HF are consistent regardless of baseline SBP.

Consistent with the larger blood pressure reductions seen in those with higher baseline SBP, empagliflozin also caused a small but

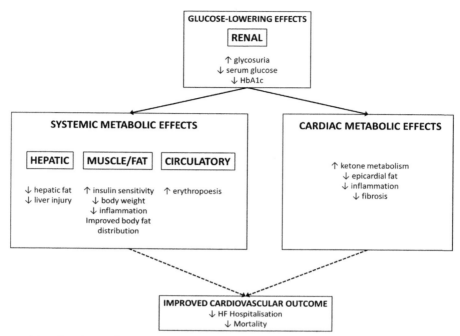

Fig. 1. Summarizing the glucose-lowering and metabolic effects of SGLT2 inhibitors that could potentially lead to improved cardiovascular outcome in patients with heart failure.

significant reduction in SBP in EMPEROR-Preserved (−1.2 mm Hg). Given the high prevalence of hypertension in HFpEF, and the higher mean SBP of the trial population compared to the HFrEF trials, a further detailed analysis of the effects related to SBP may shed light as to whether the modest blood pressure changes do indeed play a pathophysiologically important role in the mechanism of benefit in HFpEF. Interestingly, SGLT2 inhibitors have consistently shown significant reductions in left ventricular mass within 1 year that is independent of changes in blood pressure, suggesting that other mechanisms beyond blood pressure certainly play a role in the CV benefits.[32,76]

SUMMARY

So far, the mechanisms by which SGLT2 inhibitors exert benefit remain unclear. What seems certain is that it is unlikely to be just one single pathway, but rather multiple, hence their consistent benefit across a wide range of subgroups. **Fig. 1** summarizes the proposed glucose-lowering and metabolic pathways that may be involved. In a posthoc analysis of EMPA-REG Outcome, the investigators used a mediation analysis to explore what factors might drive most of the benefit of empagliflozin in the trial data.[77] It was found that the strongest association was with markers of volume status (changes in hematocrit and

hemoglobin), possibly accounting for up to 50% of the treatment effect. Changes in HbA_{1c} and fasting glucose mediated around 25% of the effect, whereas the effect of changes in BMI, blood pressure, lipids, and renal function was negligible. This is of course a posthoc analysis, but it perhaps does suggest that the diuretic effect may play a particularly important role, and this perhaps explains the early benefit seen in patients with HF.

In summary, the mechanisms of benefit of SGLT2 inhibitors remain unknown, but there is almost certainly more than 1 pathway. A key point is that the benefits in HF seem to be consistent regardless of baseline characteristics, hinting that there may indeed be multiple pathways of effect. Uncovering the mechanistic basis for the clear CV benefits of SGLT2 inhibitors remains a subject of intense research interest, and there will undoubtedly be further discovery in the near future.

CLINICS CARE POINTS

- SGLT2 inhibitors cause glucose lowering by acting on the proximal convoluted tubule of the kidney causing glycosuria.

- This lowering leads to several potentially beneficial systemic metabolic effects including action on the liver, increased erythropoiesis, and improvements in body composition.

- SGLT2 inhibitors may also improve cardiac metabolism, although further evidence is required to confirm this in patients with HF.
- It is likely that the glucose-lowering and metabolic effects of SGLT2 inhibitors contribute to the consistent CV benefits seen in patients with HF.

REFERENCES

1. Anker SD, Butler J, Filippatos G, et al. Empagliflozin in heart failure with a preserved ejection fraction. N Engl J Med 2021;385:1451–61.
2. Packer M, Anker SD, Butler J, et al. Cardiovascular and renal outcomes with empagliflozin in heart failure. N Engl J Med 2020;383:1413–24.
3. McMurray JJV, Docherty KF, Jhund PS. Dapagliflozin in patients with heart failure and reduced ejection fraction. N Engl J Med 2020;382:973.
4. Coleman RL, Gray AM, Broedl Md UC, et al. Can the cardiovascular risk reductions observed with empagliflozin in the EMPA-REG OUTCOME trial be explained by concomitant changes seen in conventional cardiovascular risk factor levels? Diabetes Obes Metab 2020;22:1151–6.
5. Lee MMY, McMurray JJV, Lorenzo-Almoros A, et al. Diabetic cardiomyopathy. Heart 2019;105:337–45.
6. Tan Y, Zhang Z, Zheng C, et al. Mechanisms of diabetic cardiomyopathy and potential therapeutic strategies: preclinical and clinical evidence. Nat Rev Cardiol 2020;17:585–607.
7. Staels B. Cardiovascular protection by sodium glucose cotransporter 2 inhibitors: potential mechanisms. Am J Med 2017;130:S30–9.
8. Tsapas A, Avgerinos I, Karagiannis T, et al. Comparative effectiveness of glucose-lowering drugs for type 2 diabetes: a systematic review and network meta-analysis. Ann Intern Med 2020;173:278–86.
9. Mordi IR, Tee A, Palmer CN, et al. Microvascular disease and heart failure with reduced and preserved ejection fraction in type 2 diabetes. ESC Heart Fail 2020;7:1168–77.
10. MacDonald MR, Petrie MC, Varyani F, et al. Impact of diabetes on outcomes in patients with low and preserved ejection fraction heart failure: an analysis of the candesartan in heart failure: assessment of reduction in mortality and morbidity (CHARM) programme. Eur Heart J 2008;29:1377–85.
11. Inzucchi SE, Docherty KF, Kober L, et al. Dapagliflozin and the incidence of type 2 diabetes in patients with heart failure and reduced ejection fraction: an exploratory analysis From DAPA-HF. Diabetes Care 2021;44:586–94.
12. Scheen AJ, Paquot N. Metabolic effects of SGLT-2 inhibitors beyond increased glucosuria: a review of the clinical evidence. Diabetes Metab 2014;40:S4–11.
13. Al Jobori H, Daniele G, Adams J, et al. Empagliflozin treatment is associated with improved beta-cell function in type 2 diabetes mellitus. J Clin Endocrinol Metab 2018;103:1402–7.
14. Lundkvist P, Pereira MJ, Kamble PG, et al. Glucagon levels during short-term SGLT2 inhibition are largely regulated by glucose changes in patients with type 2 diabetes. J Clin Endocrinol Metab 2019;104:193–201.
15. Op den Kamp YJM, de Ligt M, Dautzenberg B, et al. Effects of the SGLT2 inhibitor dapagliflozin on energy metabolism in patients with type 2 diabetes: a randomized, double-blind crossover trial. Diabetes Care 2021;44:1334–43.
16. Merovci A, Solis-Herrera C, Daniele G, et al. Dapagliflozin improves muscle insulin sensitivity but enhances endogenous glucose production. J Clin Invest 2014;124:509–14.
17. Daniele G, Xiong J, Solis-Herrera C, et al. Dapagliflozin enhances fat oxidation and ketone production in patients with type 2 diabetes. Diabetes Care 2016;39:2036–41.
18. Stanley WC, Recchia FA, Lopaschuk GD. Myocardial substrate metabolism in the normal and failing heart. Physiol Rev 2005;85:1093–129.
19. Ferrannini E, Baldi S, Frascerra S, et al. Shift to fatty substrate utilization in response to sodium-glucose Cotransporter 2 inhibition in subjects without diabetes and patients with type 2 diabetes. Diabetes 2016;65:1190–5.
20. Ferrannini E, Mark M, Mayoux E. CV protection in the EMPA-REG OUTCOME trial: a "Thrifty Substrate" hypothesis. Diabetes Care 2016;39:1108–14.
21. Singh JSS, Mordi IR, Vickneson K, et al. Dapagliflozin versus placebo on left ventricular remodeling in patients with diabetes and heart failure: the RE-FORM trial. Diabetes Care 2020;43:1356–9.
22. Pietschner R, Kolwelter J, Bosch A, et al. Effect of empagliflozin on ketone bodies in patients with stable chronic heart failure. Cardiovasc Diabetol 2021;20:219.
23. Thirunavukarasu S, Jex N, Chowdhary A, et al. Empagliflozin treatment is associated with improvements in cardiac energetics and function and reductions in myocardial cellular volume in patients with type 2 diabetes. Diabetes 2021;70:2810–22.
24. Hundertmark MJ, Agbaje OF, Coleman R, et al. Design and rationale of the EMPA-VISION trial: investigating the metabolic effects of empagliflozin in patients with heart failure. ESC Heart Fail 2021;8:2580–90.
25. Maack C, Lehrke M, Backs J, et al. Heart failure and diabetes: metabolic alterations and therapeutic interventions: a state-of-the-art review from the Translational Research Committee of the Heart Failure

Association-European Society of Cardiology. Eur Heart J 2018;39:4243–54.

26. Murphy SP, Kakkar R, McCarthy CP, et al. Inflammation in heart failure: JACC state-of-the-art review. J Am Coll Cardiol 2020;75:1324–40.

27. Curran FM, Bhalraam U, Mohan M, et al. Neutrophil-to-lymphocyte ratio and outcomes in patients with new-onset or worsening heart failure with reduced and preserved ejection fraction. ESC Heart Fail 2021;8:3168–79.

28. Aimo A, Castiglione V, Borrelli C, et al. Oxidative stress and inflammation in the evolution of heart failure: From pathophysiology to therapeutic strategies. Eur J Prev Cardiol 2020;27:494–510.

29. Heusch G, Libby P, Gersh B, et al. Cardiovascular remodelling in coronary artery disease and heart failure. Lancet 2014;383:1933–43.

30. Kolijn D, Pabel S, Tian Y, et al. Empagliflozin improves endothelial and cardiomyocyte function in human heart failure with preserved ejection fraction via reduced pro-inflammatory-oxidative pathways and protein kinase Galpha oxidation. Cardiovasc Res 2021;117:495–507.

31. Hattori S. Anti-inflammatory effects of empagliflozin in patients with type 2 diabetes and insulin resistance. Diabetol Metab Syndr 2018;10:93.

32. Brown AJM, Gandy S, McCrimmon R, et al. A randomized controlled trial of dapagliflozin on left ventricular hypertrophy in people with type two diabetes: the DAPA-LVH trial. Eur Heart J 2020;41:3421–32.

33. Requena-Ibanez JA, Santos-Gallego CG, Rodriguez-Cordero A, et al. Mechanistic Insights of Empagliflozin in Nondiabetic Patients With HFrEF: From the EMPA-TROPISM Study. JACC Heart Fail 2021;9:578–89.

34.. Correale M, Mazzeo P, Mallardi A, et al. Switch to SGLT2 inhibitors and improved endothelial function in diabetic patients with chronic heart failure. Cardiovasc Drugs Ther 2021. https://doi.org/10.1007/s10557-021-07254-3. Online ahead of print.

35. Zainordin NA, Hatta S, Mohamed Shah FZ, et al. Effects of dapagliflozin on endothelial dysfunction in type 2 diabetes with established ischemic heart disease (EDIFIED). J Endocr Soc 2020;4:bvz017.

36. Tanaka A, Shimabukuro M, Machii N, et al. Effect of empagliflozin on endothelial function in patients with type 2 diabetes and cardiovascular disease: results from the multicenter, randomized, placebo-controlled, double-blind EMBLEM trial. Diabetes Care 2019;42:e159–61.

37. Hess DA, Terenzi DC, Trac JZ, et al. SGLT2 Inhibition with empagliflozin increases circulating provascular progenitor cells in people with type 2 diabetes mellitus. Cell Metab 2019;30:609–13.

38. Lavie CJ, Alpert MA, Arena R, et al. Impact of obesity and the obesity paradox on prevalence and prognosis in heart failure. JACC Heart Fail 2013;1:93–102.

39. Aune D, Sen A, Norat T, et al. Body mass index, abdominal fatness, and heart failure incidence and mortality: a systematic review and dose-response meta-analysis of prospective studies. Circulation 2016;133:639–49.

40. Sharma A, Lavie CJ, Borer JS, et al. Meta-analysis of the relation of body mass index to all-cause and cardiovascular mortality and hospitalization in patients with chronic heart failure. Am J Cardiol 2015;115:1428–34.

41. Powell-Wiley TM, Poirier P, Burke LE, et al. American Heart Association Council on L, Cardiometabolic H, Council on C, Stroke N, Council on Clinical C, Council on E, Prevention and Stroke C. Obesity and Cardiovascular Disease: A Scientific Statement From the American Heart Association. Circulation 2021;143:e984–1010.

42.. van Woerden G, van Veldhuisen DJ, Manintveld OC, et al. Epicardial adipose tissue and outcome in heart failure with mid-range and preserved ejection fraction. Circ Heart Fail 2022;15(3):e009238. CIRCHEARTFAILURE121009238.

43. Al-Talabany S, Mordi I, Graeme Houston J, et al. Epicardial adipose tissue is related to arterial stiffness and inflammation in patients with cardiovascular disease and type 2 diabetes. BMC Cardiovasc Disord 2018;18:31.

44. Rao VN, Bush CG, Mongraw-Chaffin M, et al. Regional adiposity and risk of heart failure and mortality: the jackson heart study. J Am Heart Assoc 2021;10:e020920.

45. Rao VN, Zhao D, Allison MA, et al. Adiposity and incident heart failure and its subtypes: MESA (Multi-Ethnic Study of Atherosclerosis). JACC Heart Fail 2018;6:999–1007.

46. Pereira MJ, Eriksson JW. Emerging role of SGLT-2 inhibitors for the treatment of obesity. Drugs 2019;79:219–30.

47. Zaccardi F, Webb DR, Htike ZZ, et al. Efficacy and safety of sodium-glucose co-transporter-2 inhibitors in type 2 diabetes mellitus: systematic review and network meta-analysis. Diabetes Obes Metab 2016;18:783–94.

48. Del Prato S, Nauck M, Duran-Garcia S, et al. Long-term glycaemic response and tolerability of dapagliflozin versus a sulphonylurea as add-on therapy to metformin in patients with type 2 diabetes: 4-year data. Diabetes Obes Metab 2015;17:581–90.

49. Bolinder J, Ljunggren O, Kullberg J, et al. Effects of dapagliflozin on body weight, total fat mass, and regional adipose tissue distribution in patients with type 2 diabetes mellitus with inadequate glycemic control on metformin. J Clin Endocrinol Metab 2012;97:1020–31.

50. Diaz-Rodriguez E, Agra RM, Fernandez AL, et al. Effects of dapagliflozin on human epicardial adipose tissue: modulation of insulin resistance, inflammatory chemokine production, and differentiation ability. Cardiovasc Res 2018;114:336–46.

51. De Stefano A, Tesauro M, Di Daniele N, et al. Mechanisms of SGLT2 (Sodium-Glucose Transporter Type 2) inhibition-induced relaxation in arteries from human visceral adipose tissue. Hypertension 2021; 77:729–38.

52. Adamson C, Jhund PS, Docherty KF, et al. Efficacy of dapagliflozin in heart failure with reduced ejection fraction according to body mass index. Eur J Heart Fail 2021;23:1662–72.

53. Perrone-Filardi P, Paolillo S, Costanzo P, et al. The role of metabolic syndrome in heart failure. Eur Heart J 2015;36:2630–4.

54. Mordi IR, Lumbers RT, Palmer CNA, et al. Type 2 diabetes, metabolic traits, and risk of heart failure: a mendelian randomization study. Diabetes Care 2021;44(7):1699–705.

55. Voulgari C, Tentolouris N, Dilaveris P, et al. Increased heart failure risk in normal-weight people with metabolic syndrome compared with metabolically healthy obese individuals. J Am Coll Cardiol 2011; 58:1343–50.

56. Kaneto H, Obata A, Kimura T, et al. Beneficial effects of sodium-glucose cotransporter 2 inhibitors for preservation of pancreatic beta-cell function and reduction of insulin resistance. J Diabetes 2017;9: 219–25.

57. Ferreira JP, Verma S, Fitchett D, et al. Metabolic syndrome in patients with type 2 diabetes and atherosclerotic cardiovascular disease: a post hoc analyses of the EMPA-REG OUTCOME trial. Cardiovasc Diabetol 2020;19:200.

58. . Wang X, Ni J, Guo R, et al. SGLT2 inhibitors break the vicious circle between heart failure and insulin resistance: targeting energy metabolism. Heart Fail Rev 2022;27(3):961–80.

59. Kuchay MS, Krishan S, Mishra SK, et al. Effect of empagliflozin on liver fat in patients with type 2 diabetes and nonalcoholic fatty liver disease: a randomized controlled trial (E-LIFT Trial). Diabetes Care 2018;41:1801–8.

60. Latva-Rasku A, Honka MJ, Kullberg J, et al. The SGLT2 inhibitor dapagliflozin reduces liver fat but does not affect tissue insulin sensitivity: a randomized, double-blind, placebo-controlled study with 8-week treatment in type 2 diabetes patients. Diabetes Care 2019;42:931–7.

61. Xing B, Zhao Y, Dong B, et al. Effects of sodium-glucose cotransporter 2 inhibitors on non-alcoholic fatty liver disease in patients with type 2 diabetes: A meta-analysis of randomized controlled trials. J Diabetes Investig 2020;11:1238–47.

62. Salah HM, Pandey A, Soloveva A, et al. Relationship of nonalcoholic fatty liver disease and heart failure with preserved ejection fraction. JACC Basic Transl Sci 2021;6:918–32.

63. Verma S, McMurray JJV. SGLT2 inhibitors and mechanisms of cardiovascular benefit: a state-of-the-art review. Diabetologia 2018;61:2108–17.

64. Mordi NA, Mordi IR, Singh JS, et al. Renal and cardiovascular effects of SGLT2 inhibition in combination with loop diuretics in patients with type 2 diabetes and chronic heart failure: The RECEDE-CHF trial. Circulation 2020;142:1713–24.

65. Scholtes RA, Muskiet MHA, van Baar MJB, et al. Natriuretic effect of two weeks of dapagliflozin treatment in patients with type 2 diabetes and preserved kidney function during standardized sodium intake: results of the DAPASALT trial. Diabetes Care 2021; 44:440–7.

66. Boorsma EM, Beusekamp JC, Ter Maaten JM, et al. Effects of empagliflozin on renal sodium and glucose handling in patients with acute heart failure. Eur J Heart Fail 2021;23:68–78.

67. Hallow KM, Helmlinger G, Greasley PJ, et al. Why do SGLT2 inhibitors reduce heart failure hospitalization? A differential volume regulation hypothesis. Diabetes Obes Metab 2018;20:479–87.

68. Jensen J, Omar M, Kistorp C, et al. Effects of empagliflozin on estimated extracellular volume, estimated plasma volume, and measured glomerular filtration rate in patients with heart failure (Empire HF Renal): a prespecified substudy of a double-blind, randomised, placebo-controlled trial. Lancet Diabetes Endocrinol 2021;9:106–16.

69. Brown A, Gandy S, Mordi IR, et al. Dapagliflozin improves left ventricular myocardial longitudinal function in patients with type 2 diabetes. JACC Cardiovasc Imaging 2021;14:503–4.

70. . Ferreira JP, Anker SD, Butler J, et al. Impact of anaemia and the effect of empagliflozin in heart failure with reduced ejection fraction: findings from EMPEROR-Reduced. Eur J Heart Fail 2022;24(4): 708–15.

71. Sano M, Takei M, Shiraishi Y, et al. Increased hematocrit during sodium-glucose cotransporter 2 inhibitor therapy indicates recovery of tubulointerstitial function in diabetic kidneys. J Clin Med Res 2016; 8:844–7.

72. Fuchs FD, Whelton PK. High blood pressure and cardiovascular disease. Hypertension 2020;75: 285–92.

73. Pinho-Gomes AC, Rahimi K. Management of blood pressure in heart failure. Heart 2019;105:589–95.

74. Bohm M, Anker SD, Butler J, et al. Empagliflozin improves cardiovascular and renal outcomes in heart failure irrespective of systolic blood pressure. J Am Coll Cardiol 2021;78:1337–48.

75. Serenelli M, Bohm M, Inzucchi SE, et al. Effect of da-pagliflozin according to baseline systolic blood pressure in the Dapagliflozin and Prevention of Adverse Outcomes in Heart Failure trial (DAPA-HF). Eur Heart J 2020;41:3402–18.

76. Verma S, Mazer CD, Yan AT, et al. Effect of empagli-flozin on left ventricular mass in patients with type 2 diabetes mellitus and coronary artery disease: the EMPA-HEART CardioLink-6 randomized clinical trial. Circulation 2019;140:1693–702.

77. Inzucchi SE, Zinman B, Fitchett D, et al. How does empagliflozin reduce cardiovascular mortality? insights from a mediation analysis of the EMPA-REG OUTCOME trial. Diabetes Care 2018;41:356–63.

Renoprotective Effects of SGLT2 Inhibitors

Volker Vallon, MD[a,b,c],*

KEYWORDS

- SGLT2 inhibitor • Diabetic nephropathy • Chronic kidney disease • Tubuloglomerular feedback
- Proximal tubule • Hyperfiltration

KEY POINTS

- At the onset of therapy, SGLT2 inhibitors lower glomerular capillary pressure and filtration rate, which reduces the physical stress on the filtration barrier, the exposure of the tubular system to albumin and nephrotoxic compounds, and the oxygen demand for reabsorbing the filtered load.
- The metabolic adaptation to urinary glucose loss resembles a fasting response and includes enhanced lipolysis and hepatic formation of ketone bodies, which serve as additional fuel for the kidney.
- SGLT2 inhibitors reduce glucotoxicity in the early proximal tubule associated with improved mitochondrial function and autophagy, which helps preserve tubular transport integrity and function and, thereby, GFR in the long term.
- SGLT2 inhibitors better distribute transport work along the nephron, which may mimic systemic hypoxia at the kidney oxygen sensors in the deeper cortex and outer medulla, thereby stimulating erythropoiesis, which, together with their diuretic effect, enhances hematocrit and improves oxygen delivery to kidneys and other organs.

INTRODUCTION

Since 2008, the US Food and Drug Administration (FDA) has required proof of cardiovascular (CV) safety for new glucose-lowering therapies.[1] This also affected the development of inhibitors of the sodium-glucose cotransporter SGLT2 and produced large-scale clinical trials that were designed to confirm CV safety, but also provided, as secondary outcomes, first insights on kidney outcomes. Indeed, 3 large clinical outcome trials in patients with type 2 diabetes mellitus (T2DM) and relatively well-preserved kidney function reported that the SGLT2 inhibitors empagliflozin, dapagliflozin, and canagliflozin not only reduced the incidence of heart failure but also induced salutary effects on the kidney, including lower hazard ratios for major decline in estimated glomerular filtration rate (eGFR).[2–5] Subanalyses of these trials and systematic review and meta-analysis of multiple randomized controlled trials with various SGLT2 inhibitors indicated that the beneficial effects may extend to patients with T2DM and chronic kidney disease (CKD),[6,7] which was subsequently formally established for canagliflozin in the CREDENCE trial.[8] The DAPA-CKD trial then revealed that dapagliflozin protected the kidneys from failing relative to placebo among patients with CKD, regardless of the presence or absence of T2DM,[9] whereas a follow-up analysis suggested that the eGFR preserving effect of dapagliflozin was somewhat greater in patients with T2DM and higher HbA1c.[10] Together, the data indicate that SGLT2 inhibitors can protect the kidney independent of kidney function and T2DM, and that T2DM and/or hyperglycemia enhance the protective effects.

In the following, the kidney physiology of SGLT2 is briefly introduced, followed by the discussion of potential renoprotective effects of SGLT2 inhibitors.

[a] Division of Nephrology and Hypertension, Department of Medicine, University of California San Diego, La Jolla, CA, USA; [b] Department of Pharmacology, University of California San Diego, La Jolla, CA, USA; [c] VA San Diego Healthcare System, 3350 La Jolla Village Drive (9151), San Diego, CA 92161, USA
* VA San Diego Healthcare System, 3350 La Jolla Village Drive (9151), San Diego, CA 92161.
E-mail address: vvallon@ucsd.edu

Heart Failure Clin 18 (2022) 539–549
https://doi.org/10.1016/j.hfc.2022.03.005
1551-7136/22/© 2022 Elsevier Inc. All rights reserved.

THE PHYSIOLOGY OF SGLT2 AND ITS EXPRESSION IN THE DIABETIC KIDNEY

In euglycemia and with normal glomerular filtration rate (GFR), the proximal tubule reabsorbs almost all of the filtered glucose ($\sim$180 g/d) and thereby prevents glucose and thus valuable calories ($\sim$1/3 of the body's caloric expenditure) from being lost into the urine. The bulk of tubular glucose uptake (>90%) is mediated by high capacity SGLT2 in the "early" proximal tubule (S1/S2 segments)

(**Fig. 1**), while the glucose that escapes SGLT2 is "mopped up" by the lower capacity SGLT1 in the "late" proximal tubule (S2/S3 segments) ([11–13] and for review[14,15]) (**Fig. 2**). Glucose exits proximal tubules passively through basolateral GLUT2 (see **Fig. 1**).

The kidneys are programmed to retain the valuable energy substrate, glucose, and increase their glucose reabsorption capacity from $\sim$400 to 450 g/d to $\sim$500 to 600 g/d in patients with

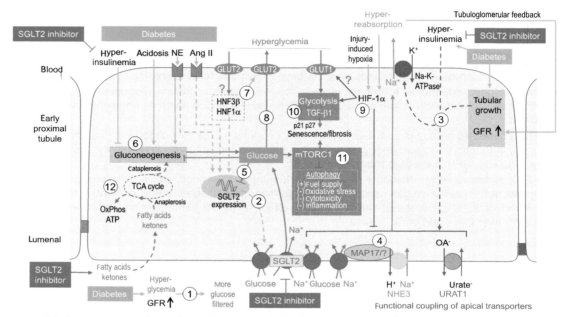

Fig. 1. Cellular processes in the early proximal tubule linked to SGLT2 and its inhibition. Hyperglycemia enhances filtered glucose and, via SGLT2, the reabsorption of glucose and Na$^+$ (1). Diabetes can increase SGLT2 expression (2) through tubular growth, angiotensin II (Ang II), sympathetic tone (norepinephrine, NE), and HNF-1α, which may respond to basolateral hyperglycemia sensed by GLUT2. Hyperinsulinemia and tubular growth upregulate proximal tubular transport systems, including SGLT2, NHE3, URAT1, and Na-K-ATPase (3). The apical transporters may be functionally coupled via scaffolding proteins, such as MAP17 (4). The resulting proximal tubular Na$^+$ retention enhances the GFR via tubuloglomerular feedback, which by increasing brush border torque can further increase transporter density in the luminal membrane. Intracellular glucose may feed back on SGLT2 upregulation (5). Diabetes, in part due to acidosis or NE, can enhance gluconeogenesis (6). Gluconeogenesis can be inhibited by tubular injury, hyperinsulinemia, and enhanced glucose uptake via SGLT2 (6). HNF-1α and HNF-3β upregulate GLUT2 (7) and thereby the basolateral exit of glucose, which maintains hyperglycemia (8). Hypoxia due to diabetes-induced hyperreabsorption or kidney injury can induce HIF-1α, which enhances basolateral glucose uptake via GLUT1, induces a metabolic shift to glycolysis, and limits apical hyperreabsorption (9). Induction of TGF-β1 and tubular growth may be particularly sensitive to basolateral glucose uptake via GLUT1 (10). Hyperinsulinemia and excessive glucose stimulate mTORC1 and attenuate autophagy (11). TGF-β1 enhances cyclin-dependent kinase inhibitors p21 and p27 and together with mTORC1 activation promotes tubular senescence, which is linked to inflammation and fibrosis. SGLT2 inhibition enhances kidney delivery of fatty acids and ketone bodies and attenuates the deleterious effects linked to hyperinsulinemia, excessive intracellular glucose, and hyperreabsorption. SGLT2 inhibition can enhance gluconeogenesis (eg, by lowering hyperinsulinemia or cytosolic glucose). Gluconeogenesis enhances removal of intermediates from TCA cycle (cataplerosis), thereby facilitating the feeding of fatty acids and ketone bodies into the TCA cycle (anaplerosis), and enhancing oxidative phosphorylation (OxPhos) and ATP generation (12). GFR, glomerular filtration rate; GLUT, facilitative glucose transporter; HIF-1α, hypoxia-inducible factor 1 alpha; HNF, hepatic nuclear factor; MAP17, 17-kDa membrane-associated protein; NHE3, Na-H-exchanger 3; OA, organic anion; TGF-β1, transforming growth factor β1; URAT1, urate transporter 1. (*Adapted from* Vallon V, Nakagawa T. Renal Tubular Handling of Glucose and Fructose in Health and Disease. Compr Physiol. 2021;12(1):2995-3044.)

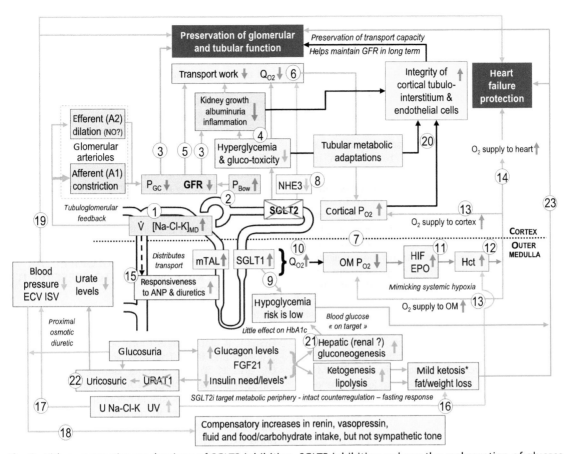

Fig. 2. Kidney protective mechanisms of SGLT2 inhibition. SGLT2 inhibition reduces the reabsorption of glucose and Na^+ in the early proximal tubule. This increases the delivery of NaCl and K ($[Na-Cl-K]_{MD}$) and fluid (V) to the macula densa, which lowers glomerular filtration rate (GFR) through the physiology of tubuloglomerular feedback (TGF) (1) and by increasing hydrostatic pressure in Bowman's space (P_{Bow}) (2). The TGF lowers GFR primarily by afferent arteriole constriction (via adenosine A1 receptor) but also by efferent arteriole dilation (via adenosine A2 receptor), which both reduce glomerular capillary pressure (P_{GC}). Lowering P_{GC} & GFR (3) and hyperglycemia (4) protects glomerular and tubular function. This includes lessening physical stress and filtration of albumin and other tubule-toxic compounds, tubular growth, and inflammation. Lowering GFR reduces tubular transport work (5), thereby lowering cortical oxygen demand (Q_{O2}) (6) and increasing cortical oxygen availability (P_{O2}) (7). Tubular transport work and toxicity are also reduced by lowering hyperglycemia and cellular SGLT2 blockade, which is also linked to inhibition of Na-H-exchanger NHE3 (8). SGLT2 inhibition shifts glucose reabsorption to downstream SGLT1, which limits glucosuria and hypoglycemia risk (9). Shifting glucose and Na^+ reabsorption to SGLT1 and medullary thick ascending limb (mTAL) increases Q_{O2} (10) and lowers P_{O2} in the outer medulla (OM) (7). which may activate hypoxia-inducible factor (HIF) and enhance erythropoietin (EPO) release (11). The resulting increase in hematocrit (Hct) (12) improves O_2 delivery to kidney medulla and cortex (13) and other organs (14). More delivery of NaCl and fluid downstream of early proximal tubule may facilitate responsiveness to atrial natriuretic peptide (ANP) and diuretics (15). The diuretic effect of SGLT2 inhibition further increases Hct (16) and reduces extracellular (ECV) and interstitial (ISV) volume and blood pressure (17). These effects are evident by compensatory upregulation of renin and vasopressin levels (18), and can help protect the failing kidney and heart (19). The increased cortical oxygen availability together with lesser tubular stress promotes the integrity of the tubular and endothelial system and preserves higher tubular transport capacity and GFR in the long term (20). The glucosuric effect lowers therapeutic and/or endogenous insulin levels and increases glucagon & FGF21 (21). This induces compensatory lipolysis, ketogenesis, and gluconeogenesis. SGLT2 inhibitors are uricosuric, potentially involving URAT1 inhibition and their glucosuric and insulin-lowering effect (22). These metabolic adaptations reduce urate levels, the hypoglycemia risk, and body and organ fat mass, which together with the resulting mild ketosis have the potential to further protect the kidney and heart (19) (23). * may contribute to reduced inflammasome activity. NO, nitric oxide; UNaClV, urinary salt excretion; UV, urinary flow rate. (*Adapted from* Vallon V. Glucose transporters in the kidney in health and disease. Pflugers Arch. 2020 Sep;472(9):1345-1370.)

T2DM and type 1 diabetes mellitus (T1DM)[14] (see **Fig. 1**). Studies in humans with T2DM[16–18] and genetic rodent models of T2DM and T1DM[16,19–21] indicate an upregulation of renal SGLT2 protein expression. Upregulation of SGLT2 expression has been linked to the overall growth and hypertrophy of the diabetic proximal tubule,[22] activation of renal sympathetic innervation[23,24] and Ang II AT1 receptors,[25] as well as the transcription factor, hepatocyte nuclear factor HNF-1α,[26] which may respond to basolateral hyperglycemia sensed through GLUT2[16] (see **Fig. 1**). The sympathetic nervous system (SNS) and HNF-1α and HNF-3β have also been implicated in the upregulation of basolateral GLUT2.[27,28] Moreover, insulin phosphorylates and increases SGLT2 activity,[29] and postprandial insulin release and hyperinsulinemia due to obesity and T2DM may increase renal SGLT2 activity to retain increased amounts of filtered glucose (see **Fig. 1**). In contrast, conditions with enhanced proximal tubule gluconeogenesis can reduce SGLT2 expression indicating negative feedback by cytosolic glucose.[30] As a consequence, renal SGLT2 expression can be unchanged or reduced in individuals with T2DM as a consequence of enhanced gluconeogenesis (eg, due to metabolic acidosis or increased sympathetic tone), or due to tubular hypoxia or injury[14] (see **Fig. 1**).

THE METABOLIC SIGNATURE OF SGLT2 INHIBITION

The logic of inhibiting SGLT2 as a therapeutic strategy in diabetes starts with the role of SGLT2 in glucose retention and maintaining hyperglycemia (see **Fig. 1**). SGLT2 inhibitors do not share the deleterious effects of other antihyperglycemic agents like an increase in body weight or hypoglycemia risk, which may offset the benefits of improving glycemic control.[31] SGLT2 inhibitors do not increase the incidence of hypoglycemia[32] because they stop lowering blood glucose once the filtered glucose load falls to the transport capacity of SGLT1 ($\sim$80 g/d).[12,14] Furthermore, SGLT2 inhibitors leave metabolic counterregulation intact, including the upregulation of gluconeogenesis in liver[32] and kidney[33] (see **Figs. 1** and **2**). Thus, SGLT2 inhibitors can improve renal and CV outcomes by preventing deleterious blood glucose highs and lows, which together cause only small changes in HbA1c.

SGLT2 inhibition shifts substrate utilization from carbohydrates to lipids, thereby reducing body fat, including visceral and subcutaneous fat[32] (see **Fig. 2**). The released free fatty acids are used for hepatic formation of ketone bodies, which provide additional energy substrates for many organs, including the kidney epithelia[34–36] (see **Figs. 1** and **2**).

It appears that spilling glucose and calories into the urine, which triggers metabolic counterregulation similar to fasting, provides unique benefits as an antihyperglycemic approach, possibly because the body's responses to environments with scarce energy resources have been intensely tested and refined during evolution for the survival of the organism.[32] The following sections discuss direct and indirect kidney protecting effects of SGLT2 inhibition that are, at least in part, independent of blood glucose lowering and have the potential to protect the kidney also in the nondiabetic setting.

SGLT2 INHIBITION LOWERS GLOMERULAR FILTRATION RATE INITIALLY TO PRESERVE IT IN LONG TERM

As the proximal tubule in the diabetic kidney grows and reabsorbs more glucose through SGLT2 and SGLT1, it also retains more sodium, followed by chloride and fluid. This lowers the delivery of Na, Cl, and K to the macula densa (MD), which, through the physiology of tubuloglomerular feedback (TGF), causes single nephron GFR (SNGFR) to increase in order to partially restore fluid and NaCl delivery to the early distal tubule and thereby urine excretion. Hyperreabsorption of fluid in the proximal tubule also reduces the tubular back pressure in Bowman space (P_{Bow}), thereby further increasing filtration pressure and SNGFR. These mechanisms form the basis for the tubular hypothesis of glomerular hyperfiltration in the diabetic kidney.[22,37]

Accordingly, inhibition of SGLT2 lowers proximal tubule hyperreabsorption in the diabetic kidney, enhances tubular back pressure and the delivery of Na, Cl, and K to the MD, and via TGF reduces glomerular hyperfiltration (see **Fig. 2**). This concept has been established by micropuncture studies in hyperfiltering diabetic rats.[37–39] Moreover, pharmacologic or genetic inhibition of SGLT2 reduced glomerular hyperfiltration in diabetic mice,[19,20,40] and the GFR-lowering effect was independent of effects on blood glucose.[20,37,39]

The GFR-lowering effect of short-term SGLT2 inhibition was confirmed in humans with T1DM and T2DM.[41] Most importantly, clinical studies have established a biphasic GFR response to SGLT2 inhibition: the initial GFR reduction is followed by long-term GFR preservation.[4,8,42–44] Moreover, after discontinuation of treatment, eGFR increased to baseline in the SGLT2 inhibitor groups.[4,42] The short-term GFR-lowering effect,[8,45,46] the long-term GFR preservation[8] as well as the reversibility after the discontinuation of the SGLT2 inhibitor[46] was confirmed in patients with T2DM and CKD level 2/3. Thus, the early rise in plasma creatinine in response to an SGLT2 inhibitor reflects a "functional and reversible" reduction in GFR, rather than kidney injury. In accordance, dapagliflozin treatment decreased urinary levels of markers of glomerular and tubular injury in patients with T2DM.[47,48] Moreover, meta-analyses of clinical studies concluded that SGLT2 inhibition induces small increases in serum creatinine but reduces the incidence of acute kidney injury.[49,50]

DOES SGLT2 INHIBITION LOWER GLOMERULAR CAPILLARY PRESSURE?

When MD cells sense an increase in luminal NaCl, the resulting TGF-induced ATP release promotes local formation of adenosine, which primarily constricts the afferent arteriole via adenosine A1 receptors[51] but can also dilate the efferent arteriole via adenosine A2 receptors[52–54] (see **Fig. 2**). Both effects are expected to lower glomerular capillary pressure (P_{GC}). Studies in mice with T1DM confirmed adenosine A1 receptor-mediated afferent arteriolar vasoconstriction in response to empagliflozin[55] (see **Fig. 2**). Micropuncture of glomerular capillaries in rats with T1DM established that the SGLT2 inhibitor ipragliflozin indeed reduced P_{GC}[38]; notably, the changes in P_{GC} and GFR were not strictly correlated. This finding cannot be explained by a sole effect on the afferent arteriole, but implied that SGLT2 inhibition constricted the afferent arteriole and also dilated the efferent arteriole,[38] and is consistent with the asymmetry of afferent and efferent arteriolar TGF responses and their consequences on GFR and P_{GC}.[38,56–58] As a consequence, SGLT2 inhibition can induce a robust reduction in P_{GC} even when GFR decreases only slightly and vice versa.[38] This may have implications in advanced CKD (GFR<30 mL/(min × 1.73 m^2)), where the initial GFR drop in response to SGLT2 inhibition can be small, but the kidney protective effect is preserved,[59] possibly due to a robust effect on the efferent arteriole and predominant reduction in P_{GC}.[38]

It was recently discovered that the MD senses an increased glucose delivery via luminal SGLT1, which then activates nitric oxide synthase 1 (NOS1), and the resulting increase in NO formation blunts the afferent arteriolar vasoconstrictor effect of TGF and thereby contributes to diabetic hyperfiltration.[40,60] Thus, the increase in MD glucose delivery in response to an SGLT2 inhibitor can activate the MD-SGLT1-NOS1 pathway and attenuate the initial GFR reduction (for details and discussion see Refs.[22,40]). Considering the close proximity of the MD to both afferent and efferent arteriole, it is also possible that the MD-SGLT1-NOS1 pathway dilates the efferent arteriole, potentially in settings with low endogenous efferent NO tone.

HOW CAN LOWERING GLOMERULAR FILTRATION RATE AND PGC PROTECT THE KIDNEY IN LONG TERM?

By reducing GFR and P_{GC} (and increasing P_{Bow}), SGLT2 inhibition reduces the physical stress on glomerular capillaries and diminishes the glomerular filtration of tubulotoxic factors (eg, albumin, growth hormones, advance glycation end products). The interaction of these factors with the tubular system requires energy and promotes hypoxia, impairs autophagy, and triggers renal oxidative stress, inflammation, and fibrosis, and thereby the development and progression of diabetic kidney disease[22,61] (see **Fig. 2**).

The preservation of cortical oxygenation appears to be critical in preserving kidney function in patients with CKD.[62] GFR is the primary determinant of renal NaCl reabsorption and, thus, of renal transport work and oxygen consumption. According to the tubular hypothesis of diabetic kidney disease, lowering single nephron glomerular hyperfiltration and thereby the oxygen-consuming transport work has the potential to preserve the integrity of the remaining nephrons and overall kidney function in the long term[22] (see **Fig. 2**). This has been proposed for blockers of angiotensin II and now for SGLT2 inhibitors, and the clinical trials provided evidence that the 2 strategies are additive and apply to patients with initial GFRs of at least 30 mL/min/ 1.73 m^2 of body-surface area.[22] Mathematical modeling predicted that SGLT2 inhibition in the diabetic kidney reduces oxygen consumption in the proximal convoluted tubule and renal cortex, in part by lowering GFR.[63,64] SGLT2 inhibition attenuated the cortical tubular expression of hypoxia-induced factor HIF-1α in a murine model of T2DM,[65] and the predicted increase in cortical O_2 pressure has been observed in a diabetic rat model using the SGLT inhibitor phlorizin[66] and with dapagliflozin in albuminuric patients with T1DM.[67]

SGLT2 inhibitors lower cortical O_2 consumption as a consequence of direct SGLT2 inhibition and the lowering of GFR[63,64,68] but may also do so as a consequence of a functional coupling of SGLT2 to other transporters in the early proximal tubule (see **Figs. 1** and **2**). This has been proposed for the Na-H-exchanger NHE3, such that pharmacologic blockade of SGLT2 partially inhibits NHE3 activity.[33,69–72] Vice versa, tubular knockdown of NHE3 reduces SGLT2 expression.[30] The effect of an SGLT2 inhibitor on NHE3 may involve the scaffolding protein MAP17,[73] phosphorylation of NHE3,[33,70,72,74] but also lower insulin levels (see **Figs. 1** and **2**). Hyperinsulinemia is known to costimulates SGLT2, NHE3, and URAT1 in the proximal tubule[14] (see **Fig. 1**). This may facilitate glomerulotubular balance during postprandial increases in GFR and insulin, but also lead to renal NaCl and urate retention in obesity and T2DM[14] (see **Figs. 1** and **2**). Coinhibition of NHE3 by SGLT2 inhibitors would enhance the natriuretic effect and lower the O_2 demand also in the nondiabetic setting.[33,70,75]

SGLT2 Inhibitors Activate Metabolic Counterregulation Similar to Fasting and Reduce Proximal Tubule Glucotoxicity

By losing glucose into the urine and activating metabolic responses similar to fasting, SGLT2 inhibitors may provide unique benefits.[32] An emerging hypothesis links this to improved autophagy in the kidney and other organs[19,76–79] (see **Fig. 1**). Empagliflozin reduced the renal accumulation of p62 in Akita mice, providing the first evidence that SGLT2 inhibition may improve autophagy in the diabetic kidney[19] (see **Fig. 1**). According to the theory, SGLT2 inhibitors reduce blood glucose and insulin levels, lower the cellular glucose availability, and stimulate a starvation-like response, which is induced independently of basal hyperglycemia. The response includes SIRT1/AMPK activation and inhibition of the AKT/mTOR1 pathway, thereby counteracting the primary pathophysiology of the proximal tubule in diabetes and overnutrition[16,35,77,79,80] and inducing autophagy, which promotes cellular defense and prosurvival mechanisms. Autophagy improves energy metabolism and fuel supply and reduces oxidative stress, cytotoxicity, and inflammation (see **Fig. 1**).

Preliminary studies in T1DM Akita mice and patients with T2DM showed that diabetes increased the urinary ratio of lactate to pyruvate, potentially indicating a metabolic shift from mitochondrial oxidation to more glycolysis, an effect reversed by SGLT2 inhibition.[81] In patients with T2DM and albuminuria, dapagliflozin increased urinary metabolites linked to mitochondrial metabolism, potentially indicating that dapagliflozin improves mitochondrial function in the diabetic kidney.[82] In accordance, scRNA-seq of proximal tubules in db/db mice indicated that although RAS blockade is more anti-inflammatory/antifibrotic, SGLT2

inhibition affected more genes related to mitochondrial function.[83] Moreover, the SGLT2 inhibitor ipragliflozin reversed the tubular and mitochondrial damage caused by high-fat diet in mice, independent of blood glucose levels.[84] Studies in nondiabetic mice provided evidence that SGLT2 inhibition causes distinct effects on kidney metabolism reflecting responses to partial NHE3 inhibition as well as urinary loss of glucose and NaCl; this included upregulation in renal gluconeogenesis and using tubular secretion of the tricarboxylic acid (TCA) cycle intermediate, alpha-ketoglutarate, to communicate to the distal nephron the need for compensatory NaCl reabsorption.[33]

SGLT2 inhibitors increase urate excretion and lower plasma urate levels; this response is related to the rise in tubular or urinary glucose delivery.[85–87] Studies in gene-targeted mouse models indicated a role for the luminal urate transporter URAT1 in the acute uricosuric effect of canagliflozin,[86] which may involve lowering of insulin levels[86,88] or other coupling mechanisms between SGLT2 and URAT1 (see **Figs. 1** and **2**).

SGLT2 Inhibition Causes More Equal Distribution of Renal Transport Work and May Mimic Systemic Hypoxia at the Renal Oxygen Sensor

The early proximal tubule is responsible for a large fraction of glomerular filtrate reabsorption and thus oxygen consumption.[63,64] SGLT2 inhibition shifts some of the glucose, NaCl, and fluid reabsorption downstream, and thereby more equally distributes the transport burden along the tubular and collecting duct system, which may help to preserve tubular function in the long term. The shift in transport to the S3 segment and thick ascending limb in the renal outer medulla, however, may reduce the O_2 availability in this region[63,64,66] (see **Fig. 2**). The increase in urinary adenosine excretion in patients with T1DM[89] and T2DM[90] in response to SGLT2 inhibition likely reflects an increase in transport work in downstream segments, which enhances ATP consumption but increases adenosine formation and release in an effort to limit medullary O_2 consumption and raise supply.[53] The increase in downstream transport work in response to SGLT2 inhibition is also limited by the reduction in blood glucose and/or GFR[63,64] (see **Fig. 2**). Moreover, we proposed that the transport shift induced by SGLT2 inhibition simulates systemic hypoxia at the oxygen sensor in the deep cortex and outer medulla of the kidney, where it stimulates HIF-1α and HIF-2α.[68] Gene knockout and pharmacologic inhibition of SGLT2 increased the renal mRNA expression of hemoxygenase 1,[19,20] a tissue-protective gene induced by HIF-1α. Upon hypoxia exposure of cells in vitro, HIF-1α and HIF-2α increase Sirt1 gene expression, which stabilizes HIF-2α signaling and EPO gene expression.[91] Thus, costimulation of HIF-1α and HIF-2α in response to SGLT2 inhibition may explain the observed increase in erythropoietin expression[33] and plasma levels.[92,93] Together with the diuretic effect, the latter may contribute to the observed modest increase in hematocrit and hemoglobin in response to SGLT2 inhibition,[94] which can improve the oxygenation of renal outer medulla and cortex and facilitate oxygen delivery to other organs (see **Fig. 2**). Mediation analyses identified the rise in hematocrit as a key determinant of renal and CV benefits of SGLT2 inhibition.[94–96] Modeling studies predict that the transport shift to the outer medulla and the natriuretic and diuretic effect of SGLT2 inhibition is in part preserved in CKD because of a high glucose load on the single nephron level (facilitated by lesser blood glucose-lowering effect), which induces paracellular sodium secretion in the proximal tubule.[68] This may contribute to the preserved protective effects of SGLT2 inhibitors in patients with CKD.

Perspectives

Much needs to be learned about the mechanisms involved in kidney protection by SGLT2 inhibitors. The SNS plays a deleterious role in the pathogenesis of CKD and is activated by classic diuretics, and this activation is absent with SGLT2 inhibitors in human and animal studies but the mechanism remains unclear.[97–102] There is also a need to better understand the consequences of SGLT2 inhibition on MD glucose delivery, their effects on glomerular hemodynamics through the efferent arteriole, and how pathophysiological conditions affect these responses. We need to further unravel the metabolic responses on the cellular level of the early proximal tubule as well as the consequences in downstream segments, including the stimulation of erythropoietin. All this information will be helpful to learn more about the patient populations that benefit from the treatment with SGLT2 inhibitors.

CLINICS CARE POINTS

- Patients must be counseled to monitor their blood pressure and diabetic patients also their blood glucose when initiating SGLT2 inhibitors.

- In the absence of an alternate cause of acute kidney injury or hemodynamic instability, the initial decline in eGFR of up to 30% after SGLT2i initiation is expected and likely due to nephroprotective reduction in intraglomerular pressure.

- Owing to the glucosuric effect of SGLT2 inhibitors and the associated increased risk of genital mycotic infections, patients must be counseled regarding maintenance of genital hygiene

- To prevent diabetic ketoacidosis, hypovolemia, and hypotension, patients must be instructed to pause taking SGLT2 inhibitors when their oral food and water intake is reduced because of underlying illness or planned surgery.

FINANCIAL SUPPORT AND SPONSORSHIP

V. Vallon is supported by NIH grants R01DK112042, R01HL142814, RF1AG061296, the UAB/UCSD O'Brien Center of Acute Kidney Injury NIH-P30DK079337, and the Department of Veterans Affairs.

ACKNOWLEDGMENTS

None.

DISCLOSURE

Over the past 24 months, V. Vallon has served as a consultant and received honoraria from Boehringer Ingelheim, Lexicon, Fibrocor, and Retrophin, and received grant support for investigator-initiated research from Astra-Zeneca, Boehringer Ingelheim, Novo-Nordisk, Kyowa-Kirin, and Janssen Pharmaceutical.

REFERENCES

1. US Food and Drug Administration. Guidance for industry: diabetes mellitus — evaluating cardiovascular risk in new antidiabetic therapies to treat type 2 diabetes. 2008. Available at: http://www.fda.gov/downloads/Drugs/GuidanceComplianceRegulatoryInformation/Guidances/ucm071627.pdf. Accessed March 26, 2019.
2. Wiviott SD, Raz I, Bonaca MP, et al. Dapagliflozin and cardiovascular outcomes in type 2 diabetes. N Engl J Med 2019;380(4):347–57.
3. Zinman B, Wanner C, Lachin JM, et al. Empagliflozin, cardiovascular outcomes, and mortality in type 2 diabetes. N Engl J Med 2015;373:2117–28.

4. Wanner C, Inzucchi SE, Lachin JM, et al. Empagliflozin and progression of kidney disease in type 2 diabetes. N Engl J Med 2016;375(4):323–34.

5. Neal B, Perkovic V, Mahaffey KW, et al. Canagliflozin and cardiovascular and renal events in type 2 diabetes. N Engl J Med 2017;377:644–57.

6. Mosenzon O, Wiviott SD, Cahn A, et al. Effects of dapagliflozin on development and progression of kidney disease in patients with type 2 diabetes: an analysis from the DECLARE-TIMI 58 randomised trial. Lancet Diabetes Endocrinol 2019;7(8): 606–17.

7. Toyama T, Neuen BL, Jun M, et al. Effect of SGLT2 inhibitors on cardiovascular, renal and safety outcomes in patients with type 2 diabetes mellitus and chronic kidney disease: A systematic review and meta-analysis. Diabetes Obes Metab 2019; 21(5):1237–50.

8. Perkovic V, Jardine MJ, Neal B, et al. Canagliflozin and renal outcomes in type 2 diabetes and nephropathy. N Engl J Med 2019;380:2295–306.

9. Heerspink HJL, Stefansson BV, Correa-Rotter R, et al. Dapagliflozin in patients with chronic kidney disease. N Engl J Med 2020;383(15):1436–46.

10. Heerspink HJL, Jongs N, Chertow GM, et al. Effect of dapagliflozin on the rate of decline in kidney function in patients with chronic kidney disease with and without type 2 diabetes: a prespecified analysis from the DAPA-CKD trial. Lancet Diabetes Endocrinol 2021;9(11):743–54.

11. Vallon V, Platt KA, Cunard R, et al. SGLT2 mediates glucose reabsorption in the early proximal tubule. J Am Soc Nephrol 2011;22:104–12.

12. Rieg T, Masuda T, Gerasimova M, et al. Increase in SGLT1-mediated transport explains renal glucose reabsorption during genetic and pharmacological SGLT2 inhibition in euglycemia. Am J Physiol Renal Physiol 2014;306(2):F188–93.

13. Gorboulev V, Schurmann A, Vallon V, et al. Na(+)-D-glucose cotransporter SGLT1 is pivotal for intestinal glucose absorption and glucose-dependent incretin secretion. Diabetes 2012;61(1):187–96.

14. Vallon V. Glucose transporters in the kidney in health and disease. Pflugers Arch 2020;472(9):1345–70.

15. Wright EM, Loo DD, Hirayama BA. Biology of human sodium glucose transporters. Physiol Rev 2011;91(2):733–94.

16. Umino H, Hasegawa K, Minakuchi H, et al. High basolateral glucose increases sodium-glucose cotransporter 2 and reduces sirtuin-1 in renal tubules through glucose transporter-2 detection. Sci Rep 2018;8(1):6791.

17. Rahmoune H, Thompson PW, Ward JM, et al. Glucose transporters in human renal proximal tubular cells isolated from the urine of patients with non-insulin-dependent diabetes. Diabetes 2005;54(12):3427–34.

18. Wang XX, Levi J, Luo Y, et al. SGLT2 expression is increased in human diabetic nephropathy: SGLT2 inhibition decreases renal lipid accumulation, inflammation and the development of nephropathy in diabetic mice. J Biol Chem 2017;292:5335–48.

19. Vallon V, Gerasimova M, Rose MA, et al. SGLT2 inhibitor empagliflozin reduces renal growth and albuminuria in proportion to hyperglycemia and prevents glomerular hyperfiltration in diabetic Akita mice. Am J Physiol Renal Physiol 2014;306(2):F194–204.

20. Vallon V, Rose M, Gerasimova M, et al. Knockout of Na-glucose transporter SGLT2 attenuates hyperglycemia and glomerular hyperfiltration but not kidney growth or injury in diabetes mellitus. Am J Physiol Ren Physiol 2013;304(2):F156–67.

21. Wen L, Zhang Z, Peng R, et al. Whole transcriptome analysis of diabetic nephropathy in the db/db mouse model of type 2 diabetes. J Cell Biochem 2019;120(10):17520–33.

22. Vallon V, Thomson SC. The tubular hypothesis of nephron filtration and diabetic kidney disease. Nat Rev Nephrol 2020;16(6):317–36.

23. Katsurada K, Nandi SS, Sharma NM, et al. Enhanced expression and function of renal SGLT2 (Sodium-Glucose Cotransporter 2) in heart failure: role of renal nerves. Circ Heart Fail 2021; 14(12):e008365.

24. de Oliveira TL, Lincevicius GS, Shimoura CG, et al. Effects of renal denervation on cardiovascular, metabolic and renal functions in streptozotocin-induced diabetic rats. Life Sci 2021;278:119534.

25. Osorio H, Bautista R, Rios A, et al. Effect of treatment with losartan on salt sensitivity and SGLT2 expression in hypertensive diabetic rats. Diabetes Res Clin Pract 2009;86(3):e46–9.

26. Freitas HS, Anhe GF, Melo KF, et al. Na(+)-glucose transporter-2 messenger ribonucleic acid expression in kidney of diabetic rats correlates with glycemic levels: involvement of hepatocyte nuclear factor-1alpha expression and activity. Endocrinology 2008;149(2):717–24.

27. Freitas HS, Schaan BD, David-Silva A, et al. SLC2A2 gene expression in kidney of diabetic rats is regulated by HNF-1alpha and HNF-3beta. Mol Cell Endocrinol 2009;305(1–2):63–70.

28. Chhabra KH, Morgan DA, Tooke BP, et al. Reduced renal sympathetic nerve activity contributes to elevated glycosuria and improved glucose tolerance in hypothalamus-specific Pomc knockout mice. Mol Metab 2017;6(10):1274–85.

29. Ghezzi C, Wright EM. Regulation of the human Na+ dependent glucose cotransporter hSGLT2. Am J Physiol Cell Physiol 2012;303:C348–54.

30. Onishi A, Fu Y, Darshi M, et al. Effect of renal tubule-specific knockdown of the Na(+)/H(+) exchanger NHE3 in Akita diabetic mice. Am J Physiol Ren Physiol 2019;317:F419–34.

31. Khunti K, Davies M, Majeed A, et al. Hypoglycemia and risk of cardiovascular disease and all-cause mortality in insulin-treated people with type 1 and type 2 diabetes: a cohort study. Diabetes Care 2015;38(2):316–22.

32. Vallon V, Thomson SC. Targeting renal glucose reabsorption to treat hyperglycaemia: the pleiotropic effects of SGLT2 inhibition. Diabetologia 2017; 60(2):215–25.

33. Onishi A, Fu Y, Patel R, et al. A role for tubular Na(+)/H(+) exchanger NHE3 in the natriuretic effect of the SGLT2 inhibitor empagliflozin. Am J Physiol Ren Physiol 2020;319(4):F712–28.

34. Qiu H, Novikov A, Vallon V. Ketosis and diabetic ketoacidosis in response to SGLT2 inhibitors: Basic mechanisms and therapeutic perspectives. Diabetes Metab Res Rev 2017;33:5.

35. Tomita I, Kume S, Sugahara S, et al. SGLT2 inhibition mediates protection from diabetic kidney disease by promoting ketone body-induced mTORC1 Inhibition. Cell Metab 2020;32(3):404–19.

36. Ferrannini E, Mark M, Mayoux E. CV Protection in the EMPA-REG OUTCOME trial: a "Thrifty Substrate" Hypothesis. Diabetes Care 2016;39(7):1108–14.

37. Vallon V, Richter K, Blantz RC, et al. Glomerular hyperfiltration in experimental diabetes mellitus: potential role of tubular reabsorption. J Am Soc Nephrol 1999;10(12):2569–76.

38. Thomson SC, Vallon V. Effects of SGLT2 inhibitor and dietary NaCl on glomerular hemodynamics assessed by micropuncture in diabetic rats. Am J Physiol Ren Physiol 2021;320:F761–77.

39. Thomson SC, Rieg T, Miracle C, et al. Acute and chronic effects of SGLT2 blockade on glomerular and tubular function in the early diabetic rat. Am J Physiol Regul Integr Comp Physiol 2012;302(1): R75–83.

40. Song P, Huang W, Onishi A, et al. Knockout of Na-glucose-cotransporter SGLT1 mitigates diabetes-induced upregulation of nitric oxide synthase-1 in macula densa and glomerular hyperfiltration. Am J Physiol Ren Physiol 2019;317:F207–17.

41. Vallon V, Verma S. Effects of SGLT2 inhibitors on kidney and cardiovascular function. Annu Rev Physiol 2021;83:503–28.

42. Perkovic V, Jardine M, Vijapurkar U, et al. Renal effects of canagliflozin in type 2 diabetes mellitus. Curr Med Res Opin 2015;31(12):2219–31.

43. Heerspink HJ, Desai M, Jardine M, et al. Canagliflozin slows progression of renal function decline independently of glycemic effects. J Am Soc Nephrol 2018;28:368–75.

44. Kohan DE, Fioretto P, Johnsson K, et al. The effect of dapagliflozin on renal function in patients with type 2 diabetes. J Nephrol 2016;29(3):391–400.

45. Yale JF, Bakris G, Cariou B, et al. Efficacy and safety of canagliflozin in subjects with type 2 diabetes and chronic kidney disease. Diabetes Obes Metab 2013;15(5):463–73.

46. Barnett AH, Mithal A, Manassie J, et al. Efficacy and safety of empagliflozin added to existing anti-diabetes treatment in patients with type 2 diabetes and chronic kidney disease: a randomised, double-blind, placebo-controlled trial. Lancet Diabetes Endocrinol 2014;2(5):369–84.

47. Dekkers CCJ, Petrykiv S, Laverman GD, et al. Effects of the SGLT-2 inhibitor dapagliflozin on glomerular and tubular injury markers. Diabetes Obes Metab 2018;20(8):1988–93.

48. Satirapoj B, Korkiatpitak P, Supasyndh O. Effect of sodium-glucose cotransporter 2 inhibitor on proximal tubular function and injury in patients with type 2 diabetes: a randomized controlled trial. Clin Kidney J 2019;12(3):326–32.

49. Gilbert RE, Thorpe KE. Acute kidney injury with sodium-glucose co-transporter-2 inhibitors: a meta-analysis of cardiovascular outcome trials. Diabetes Obes Metab 2019;21(8):1996–2000.

50. Neuen BL, Young T, Heerspink HJL, et al. SGLT2 inhibitors for the prevention of kidney failure in patients with type 2 diabetes: a systematic review and meta-analysis. Lancet Diabetes Endocrinol 2019;7(11):845–54.

51. Vallon V, Unwin R, Inscho EW, et al. Extracellular nucleotides and P2 receptors in renal function. Physiol Rev 2020;100(1):211–69.

52. Ren Y, Garvin JL, Carretero OA. Efferent arteriole tubuloglomerular feedback in the renal nephron. Kidney Int 2001;59(1):222–9.

53. Vallon V, Muhlbauer B, Osswald H. Adenosine and kidney function. Physiol Rev 2006;86(3):901–40.

54. Ren Y, Garvin JL, Liu R, et al. Possible mechanism of efferent arteriole (Ef-Art) tubuloglomerular feedback. Kidney Int 2007;71(9):861–6.

55. Kidokoro K, Cherney DZI, Bozovic A, et al. Evaluation of glomerular hemodynamic function by empagliflozin in diabetic mice using in vivo imaging. Circulation 2019;140(4):303–15.

56. Thomson S, Vallon V, Blantz RC. Asymmetry of tubuloglomerular feedback effector mechanism with respect to ambient tubular flow. Am J Physiol 1996;271(6 Pt 2):F1123–30.

57. Blantz RC, Vallon V. Tubuloglomerular feedback responses of the downstream efferent resistance: unmasking a role for adenosine? Kidney Int 2007; 71(9):837–9.

58. Schnermann J, Briggs JP. Single nephron comparison of the effect of loop of Henle flow on filtration rate and pressure in control and angiotensin II-infused rats. Miner Electrolyte Metab 1989;15(3): 103–7.

59. Bakris G, Oshima M, Mahaffey KW, et al. Effects of Canagliflozin in patients with Baseline eGFR <30 ml/min per 1.73 m(2): subgroup analysis of the

randomized CREDENCE Trial. Clin J Am Soc Nephrol 2020;15(12):1705–14.

60. Zhang J, Wei J, Jiang S, et al. Macula densa SGLT1-NOS1-TGF pathway – a new mechanism for glomerular hyperfiltration during hyperglycemia. J Am Soc Nephrol 2019;30(4):578–93.

61. Vallon V, Komers R. Pathophysiology of the diabetic kidney. Compr Physiol 2011;1:1175–232.

62. Pruijm M, Milani B, Pivin E, et al. Reduced cortical oxygenation predicts a progressive decline of renal function in patients with chronic kidney disease. Kidney Int 2018;93:932–40.

63. Layton AT, Vallon V, Edwards A. Modeling oxygen consumption in the proximal tubule: effects of NHE and SGLT2 inhibition. Am J Physiol Ren Physiol 2015;308(12):F1343–57.

64. Layton AT, Vallon V, Edwards A. Predicted consequences of diabetes and SGLT inhibition on transport and oxygen consumption along a rat nephron. Am J Physiol Ren Physiol 2016;310:F1269–83.

65. Bessho R, Takiyama Y, Takiyama T, et al. Hypoxia-inducible factor-1alpha is the therapeutic target of the SGLT2 inhibitor for diabetic nephropathy. Sci Rep 2019;9(1):14754.

66. Neill O, Fasching A, Pihl L, et al. Acute SGLT inhibition normalizes oxygen tension in the renal cortex but causes hypoxia in the renal medulla in anaesthetized control and diabetic rats. Am J Physiol Ren Physiol 2015;309:F227–34.

67. Laursen JC, Sondergaard-Heinrich N, de Melo JML, et al. Acute effects of dapagliflozin on renal oxygenation and perfusion in type 1 diabetes with albuminuria: A randomised, double-blind, placebo-controlled crossover trial. EClinicalMedicine 2021;37:100895.

68. Layton AT, Vallon V. SGLT2 inhibition in a kidney with reduced nephron number: modeling and analysis of solute transport and metabolism. Am J Physiol Ren Physiol 2018;314:F969–84.

69. Pessoa TD, Campos LC, Carraro-Lacroix L, et al. Functional role of glucose metabolism, osmotic stress, and sodium-glucose cotransporter isoform-mediated transport on Na+/H+ exchanger isoform 3 activity in the renal proximal tubule. J Am Soc Nephrol 2014;25(25):2028–39.

70. Borges-Junior FA, Silva Dos Santos D, Benetti A, et al. Empagliflozin inhibits proximal tubule NHE3 activity, preserves GFR, and restores euvolemia in nondiabetic rats with induced heart failure. J Am Soc Nephrol 2021;32:1616–29.

71. Huang W, Patel R, Onishi A, et al. Tubular NHE3 is a determinant of the acute natriuretic and chronic blood pressure lowering effect of the SGLT2 inhibitor empagliflozin. FASEB J 2018;32(Supplement No 1):620-617.

72. Fu Y, Gerasimova M, Mayoux E, et al. SGLT2 inhibitor empagliflozin increases renal NHE3 phosphorylation in diabetic Akita mice: possible implications for the prevention of glomerular hyperfiltration. Diabetes 2014;63(supplement 1):A132.

73. Coady MJ, El TA, Santer R, et al. MAP17 is a necessary activator of renal Na+/Glucose cotransporter SGLT2. J Am Soc Nephrol 2017;28:85–93.

74. Masuda T, Watanabe Y, Fukuda K, et al. Unmasking a sustained negative effect of SGLT2 inhibition on body fluid volume in the rat. Am J Physiol Ren Physiol 2018;315:F653–64.

75. Layton AT, Laghmani K, Vallon V, et al. Solute transport and oxygen consumption along the nephrons: effects of Na+ transport inhibitors. Am J Physiol Ren Physiol 2016;311(6):F1217–29.

76. Fukushima K, Kitamura S, Tsuji K, et al. Sodium-glucose cotransporter 2 inhibitors work as a "Regulator" of autophagic activity in overnutrition diseases. Front Pharmacol 2021;12:761842.

77. Fukushima K, Kitamura S, Tsuji K, et al. Sodium glucose co-transporter 2 inhibitor ameliorates autophagic flux impairment on renal proximal tubular cells in obesity mice. Int J Mol Sci 2020;21(11):4054.

78. Packer M. SGLT2 inhibitors produce cardiorenal benefits by promoting adaptive cellular reprogramming to induce a state of fasting mimicry: a paradigm shift in understanding their mechanism of action. Diabetes Care 2020;43(3):508–11.

79. Lee YH, Kim SH, Kang JM, et al. Empagliflozin attenuates diabetic tubulopathy by improving mitochondrial fragmentation and autophagy. Am J Physiol Ren Physiol 2019;317(4):F767–80.

80. Vallon V. The proximal tubule in the pathophysiology of the diabetic kidney. Am J Physiol Regul Integr Comp Physiol 2011;300(5):R1009–22.

81. Darshi M, Onishi A, Kim JJ, et al. Metabolic reprogramming in diabetic kidney disease can be restored via SGLT2 inhibition. J Am Soc Nephrol 2017;439:439 (Abstract).

82. Mulder S, Heerspink HJL, Darshi M, et al. Effects of dapagliflozin on urinary metabolites in people with type 2 diabetes. Diabetes Obes Metab 2019;21(11):2422–8.

83. Wu J, Sun Z, Yang S, et al. Profiling of kidney transcriptome at the single-cell level reveals a distinct response of proximal tubular cells to SGLT2 inhibitor and angiotensin receptor blocker treatment in diabetic mice. Mol Ther 2021. https://doi.org/10.1016/j.ymthe.2021.10.013. S1525-0016(21)00520-7.

84. Takagi S, Li J, Takagaki Y, et al. Ipragliflozin improves mitochondrial abnormalities in renal tubules induced by a high-fat diet. J Diabetes Investig 2018;9(5):1025–32.

85. Lytvyn Y, Skrtic M, Yang GK, et al. Glycosuria-mediated urinary uric acid excretion in patients

with uncomplicated type 1 diabetes mellitus. Am J Physiol Ren Physiol 2015;308(2):F77–83.

86. Novikov A, Fu Y, Huang W, et al. SGLT2 inhibition and renal urate excretion: role of luminal glucose, GLUT9, and URAT1. Am J Physiol Ren Physiol 2019;316(1):F173–85.

87. Chino Y, Samukawa Y, Sakai S, et al. SGLT2 inhibitor lowers serum uric acid through alteration of uric acid transport activity in renal tubule by increased glycosuria. Biopharm Drug Dispos 2014;35(7): 391–404.

88. Toyoki D, Shibata S, Kuribayashi-Okuma E, et al. Insulin stimulates uric acid reabsorption via regulating urate transporter 1 and ATP-binding cassette subfamily G member 2. Am J Physiol Ren Physiol 2017;313(3):F826–34.

89. Rajasekeran H, Lytvyn Y, Bozovic A, et al. Urinary adenosine excretion in type 1 diabetes. Am J Physiol Ren Physiol 2017;313(2):F184–91.

90. van Bommel EJM, Muskiet MHA, van Baar MJB, et al. The renal hemodynamic effects of the SGLT2 inhibitor dapagliflozin are caused by postglomerular vasodilatation rather than preglomerular vasoconstriction in metformin-treated patients with type 2 diabetes in the randomized, double-blind RED trial. Kidney Int 2020;97(1): 202–12.

91. Chen R, Dioum EM, Hogg RT, et al. Hypoxia increases sirtuin 1 expression in a hypoxiainducible factor-dependent manner. J Biol Chem 2011;286(16):13869–78.

92. Mazer CD, Hare GMT, Connelly PW, et al. Effect of empagliflozin on erythropoietin levels, iron stores and red blood cell morphology in patients with type 2 diabetes and coronary artery disease. Circulation 2020;141(8):704–7.

93. Ghanim H, Abuaysheh S, Hejna J, et al. Dapagliflozin suppresses hepcidin and increases erythropoiesis. J Clin Endocrinol Metab 2020;105(4): dgaa057.

94. Inzucchi SE, Zinman B, Fitchett D, et al. How does empagliflozin reduce cardiovascular mortality? insights from a mediation analysis of the EMPA-REG OUTCOME trial. Diabetes Care 2018;41(2): 356–63.

95. Li J, Neal B, Perkovic V, et al. Mediators of the effects of canagliflozin on kidney protection in patients with type 2 diabetes. Kidney Int 2020;98(3): 769–77.

96. Li J, Woodward M, Perkovic V, et al. Mediators of the effects of canagliflozin on heart failure in patients with type 2 diabetes. JACC Heart Fail 2020; 8(1):57–66.

97. Verma S. Are the cardiorenal benefits of SGLT2 inhibitors due to inhibition of the sympathetic nervous system? JACC Basic Transl Sci 2020;5(2): 180–2.

98. Wan N, Fujisawa Y, Kobara H, et al. Effects of an SGLT2 inhibitor on the salt sensitivity of blood pressure and sympathetic nerve activity in a nondiabetic rat model of chronic kidney disease. Hypertens Res 2020;43(6):492–9.

99. Matthews VB, Elliot RH, Rudnicka C, et al. Role of the sympathetic nervous system in regulation of the sodium glucose cotransporter 2. J Hypertens 2017;35(10):2059–68.

100. Chiba Y, Yamada T, Tsukita S, et al. Dapagliflozin, a Sodium-Glucose Co-Transporter 2 inhibitor, acutely reduces energy expenditure in BAT via neural signals in mice. PLoS One 2016;11(3):e0150756.

101. Herat LY, Magno AL, Rudnicka C, et al. SGLT2 inhibitor-induced sympathoinhibition: a novel mechanism for cardiorenal protection. JACC Basic Transl Sci 2020;5(2):169–79.

102. Jordan J, Tank J, Heusser K, et al. The effect of empagliflozin on muscle sympathetic nerve activity in patients with type II diabetes mellitus. J Am Soc Hypertens 2017;11(9):604–12.

SGLT2 Inhibitors in Type 2 Diabetes Mellitus

Giulia Ferrannini, MD[a], Gianluigi Savarese, MD, PhD[a,b], Francesco Cosentino, MD, PhD[a,b],*

KEYWORDS

- Sodium-glucose cotransporter 2 inhibitors • Type 2 diabetes • Cardiovascular outcomes
- Heart failure

KEY POINTS

- Sodium-glucose cotransporter 2 inhibitors are a class of glucose-lowering drugs, primarily used in patients with type 2 diabetes, which were tested in cardiovascular outcome trials following guidance from international medicines agencies.
- Results from cardiovascular outcome trials showed that sodium-glucose cotransporter 2 inhibitors are safe and noninferior compared with placebo on top of standard medical care.
- The most consistent cardiovascular effect of sodium-glucose cotransporter 2 inhibitors in cardiovascular outcome trials was the benefit on heart failure–related events, including first and recurrent hospitalization, and cardiovascular death.
- Real-world observations substantially confirmed trials' findings.
- Sodium-glucose cotransporter 2 inhibitors gained the attention of the scientific community because of their striking clinical benefit, and the investigation of the underlying mechanisms granting such benefit is continuously engaging researchers all over the world.

HISTORY OF SODIUM-GLUCOSE TRANSPORTER INHIBITORS

The first discovered sodium-glucose transporter (SGLT) inhibitor was phlorizin, a glucoside found in the root bark of apple trees, isolated by de Konink in 1836.[1] In 1885, von Mering observed that intravenous administration of phlorizin caused glucosuria and consequently had a diuretic effect,[2] prompting clinical research in different settings including renal function, metabolism, sarcoma, and nephritis.[3] The inhibiting action of phlorizin on the transporter, causing glucose reabsorption in the renal proximal tubule and in the intestine, was observed in vitro in the second half of the twentieth century; two main isoforms were then identified, "intestinal" (SGLT1) and "kidney" (SGLT2).[4–7] In light of the observation that phlorizin normalized glucose levels and decreased insulin resistance in diabetic rats, a group of researchers from Japan synthetized the first oral phlorizin-like compound.[8–10] In the last 20 years, pharmacologic industries have commercialized several products, most with SGLT2 selectivity (**Table 1**).[11]

GUIDANCE FOR CARDIOVASCULAR OUTCOME TRIALS IN TYPE 2 DIABETES

In 2008, after the observation that marketed antidiabetic agents increased the risk of cardiovascular events and mortality, the Food and Drug Administration and the European Medicines Agency issued a guidance to the pharmaceutical industries, stating that "concerns about cardiovascular risk should be more thoroughly addressed during drug development."[12,13] Trials for SGLT2i made no exception and were thus designed as cardiovascular outcome trials (CVOTs), assessing cardiovascular efficacy

[a] Division of Cardiology, Department of Medicine, Solna, Karolinska Institutet, Norrbacka S1:02, Stockholm SE 17177, Sweden; [b] Heart, Vascular and Neuro Theme, Department of Cardiology, Karolinska University Hospital, Anna Steckséns gata 41, 171 64 Solna, Sweden
* Corresponding author. Division of Cardiology, Department of Medicine, Solna, Karolinska Institutet, Norrbacka S1:02, Stockholm SE 17177, Sweden.
E-mail address: francesco.cosentino@ki.se

Heart Failure Clin 18 (2022) 551–559
https://doi.org/10.1016/j.hfc.2022.03.009
1551-7136/22/© 2022 The Author(s). Published by Elsevier Inc. This is an open access article under the CC BY license (http://creativecommons.org/licenses/by/4.0/).

Table 1
Characteristics of currently approved sodium-glucose cotransporter 2 inhibitors

Name of the Drug	Available Tablet Doses	Indications	Renal Function[b]	Approvals[a]
Canagliflozin	100 mg, 300 mg	T2DM	Initiation contraindicated if eGFR <30	EMA (2013), FDA (2013), Australia (2013)
Dapagliflozin	5 mg, 10 mg	T2DM, HF, CKD (FDA only)	Initiation contraindicated if eGFR <25	EMA (2012), FDA (2014)
Empagliflozin	10 mg, 25 mg	T2DM, HF	In T2DM: not recommended if eGFR <45 (EMA)/30 (FDA) In HF: not recommended if eGFR <20	EMA (2014), FDA (2014)
Ertugliflozin	5 mg, 15 mg	T2DM	EMA: initiation not recommended if eGFR <45 FDA: initiation not recommended if eGFR <30	EMA (2018), FDA (2019)
Sotagliflozin	200 mg	T1DM	EMA: initiation not recommended if eGFR <60	EMA 2019
Ipragliflozin	25 mg, 50 mg	T2DM	Not stated	Japan 2014, Republic of Korea and Thailand 2015, Russia 2019
Luseogliflozin	2.5 mg, 5 mg	T2DM	Not recommended if GFR <60	Japan 2014
Tofogliflozin	20 mg	T2DM	Not stated	Japan 2014
Remogliflozin	100 mg	T2DM, NAFLD	Not stated	India 2019

Abbreviations: CKD, chronic kidney disease; eGFR, estimated glomerular filtration rate; EMA, European Medicines Agency; FDA, Food and Drug Administration; HF, heart failure; NAFLD, nonalcoholic fatty liver disease; T1DM, type 1 diabetes mellitus; T2DM, type 2 diabetes mellitus.
[a] Refers to first approval in type 2 diabetes.
[b] eGFR is in mL/min/1.73 m^2.

and safety, with a composite end point of three-point major adverse cardiovascular events (3P-MACE) including first of cardiovascular death, nonfatal myocardial infarction, and nonfatal stroke. Therefore, these trials included patients at high cardiovascular risk or with established cardiovascular disease (CVD), with varying proportions of heart failure (HF) at baseline and generally increased risk to develop HF-related events (**Table 2**).

CARDIOVASCULAR OUTCOME TRIALS IN PATIENTS WITH TYPE 2 DIABETES MELLITUS: A MAJOR BREAKTHROUGH

The Empagliflozin, Cardiovascular Outcomes, and Mortality in Type 2 Diabetes (EMPA-REG OUTCOME) trial was the landmark trial for this class of drugs: 7020 patients with type 2 diabetes mellitus (T2DM) and a history of a previous cardiovascular event were randomized to either empagliflozin (10 or 25 mg) or placebo on top of standard care (**Table 3**).[14] Although designed as a noninferiority trial for 3P-MACE, in EMPA-REG OUTCOME empagliflozin reduced the risk of not only this primary outcome (hazard ratio [HR], 0.86; 95% confidence interval [CI], 0.74–0.99; $P = .0038$), but also of all-cause mortality (32% relative risk reduction), cardiovascular mortality (38% relative risk reduction), and HF hospitalizations (HHF; 35% relative risk reduction) over a median follow-up of 3.1 years. The separation of the Kaplan-Meier curves for either HHF or cardiovascular death occurred early

Table 2
Baseline characteristics of the populations of cardiovascular outcome trials on sodium-glucose cotransporter 2 inhibitors

	EMPA-REG OUTCOME	DECLARE-TIMI 58	CANVAS Program	CREDENCE	VERTIS-CV
Number of participants	7020	17,160	10,142	4401	8246
Drug	Empagliflozin	Dapagliflozin	Canagliflozin	Canagliflozin	Ertugliflozin
Women, %	28.5	37.4	35.8	33.9	30.0
HbA$_{1c}$, mean	8.1	8.3	8.2	8.3	8.2
Diabetes duration, mean (SD), y	10 (in >57% participants)	11.8 (7.8)	13.5 (7.8)	15.8 (8.6)	13.0 (8.3)
Established ASCVD, %	100	40.6	65.6	50.4	100
Heart failure, %	10.1	10.0	14.4	14.8	23.7
eGFR <60 mL/min/m^2, %	25.9	7.4	20.1	59.8	21.9

Abbreviations: ASCVD, atherosclerotic cardiovascular disease; CANVAS, CANagliflozin cardioVascular Assessment Study; CREDENCE, Canagliflozin and Renal Events in Diabetes with Established Nephropathy Clinical Evaluation; DECLARE-TIMI 58, Dapagliflozin Effect on Cardiovascular Events–Thrombolysis in Myocardial Infarction 58; eGFR, estimated glomerular filtration rate; EMPA-REG OUTCOME, Empagliflozin, Cardiovascular Outcomes, and Mortality in Type 2 Diabetes; HbA$_{1c}$, glycated hemoglobin; SD, standard deviation; VERTIS-CV, eValuation of ERTugliflozin effIcacy and Safety CardioVascular outcomes trial.

in the trial, leading to a number needed to treat to prevent one such event of 35 over 3 years.[15] The effect of empagliflozin was consistent in patients with and without HF at baseline and across subgroups with different glucose-lowering drugs and HF treatments.[15] Moreover, in patients without HF at baseline, empagliflozin consistently reduced the risk of cardiovascular death and HHF irrespective of their baseline HF risk.[16] In a post hoc analysis of the 221 patients who experienced at least one HHF after randomization in EMPA-REG OUTCOME, the number of adjudicated clinical events (second events of HF rehospitalization, HF rehospitalization or cardiovascular death, HF rehospitalization or all-cause death) within 30, 45, 60, and 90 days from the admission date of first HHF were compared in the empagliflozin (126 patients) versus placebo (95 patients) groups.[17] After 30 days, the rates of readmission were nearly two-fold higher in patients who received placebo compared with empagliflozin.[17] Essentially, empagliflozin emerged as a potential treatment of HF, because its effect was in the same magnitude of that of established HF treatment (eg, enalapril and eplerenone).[18,19]

In the Dapagliflozin Effect on Cardiovascular Events–Thrombolysis in Myocardial Infarction 58 (DECLARE-TIMI 58) trial, where 17,160 patients with T2DM and with or at risk of atherosclerotic CVD (ASCVD) were randomized to dapagliflozin or placebo on top of standard therapy, dapagliflozin was not superior to placebo as regards 3P-MACE (HR, 0.93; 95% CI, 0.84–1.03), but the risk of the coprimary outcome of cardiovascular death or HHF was significantly reduced in the

dapagliflozin group, driven mainly by a 27% reduction in risk of HHF.[20] The effect of dapagliflozin on this composite outcome was greater in patients with a previous myocardial infarction, in patients with higher levels of N-terminal pro–brain natriuretic peptide and high-sensitivity troponin T, but independent of T2DM duration.[21–23] As regards baseline HF status, the risk reduction in HHF conferred by dapagliflozin treatment was consistent in patients with and without prior HF, but the risk of cardiovascular death was reduced only in patients with HF with reduced ejection fraction.[24]

Canagliflozin was tested in the CANagliflozin cardioVascular Assessment Study (CANVAS) Programme, a combined analysis of two double-blind placebo-controlled trials enrolling a total of 10,142 patients with T2DM who were randomized to canagliflozin versus placebo on top of optimal medical care.[25] Among them, 66% had established CVD and 34% had high cardiovascular risk.[26] Canagliflozin was superior to placebo, significantly reducing the risk of 3P-MACE by 14%, and the risk of HHF by 33%.[26] A post hoc analysis suggested that the benefit of canagliflozin on cardiovascular death or HHF may be greater in patients with a history of HF (HR, 0.61; 95% CI, 0.46–0.80), who constituted 14% of the whole trial population, compared with those without HF at baseline (HR, 0.87; 95% CI, 0.72–1.06; P value for interaction 0.021), with no additional safety concerns.[27] The efficacy of canagliflozin was consistent across different body mass index strata[28] and renal function.[29]

Table 3
Summary results of cardiovascular outcomes in cardiovascular outcome trials on sodium-glucose cotransporter 2 inhibitors

	EMPA-REG OUTCOME	DECLARE-TIMI 58	CANVAS Program	CREDENCE	VERTIS-CV	Overall[a]
3P-MACE	0.86 (0.74–0.99)	0.93 (0.84–1.03)	0.86 (0.75–0.97)	0.80 (0.67–0.95)	0.99 (0.88–1.12)	0.90 (0.85–0.95)
HHF	0.65 (0.50–0.85)	0.73 (0.61–0.88)	0.67 (0.52–0.87)	0.61 (0.47–0.80)	0.70 (0.54–0.90)	0.68 (0.61–0.76)
CV death	0.62 (0.49–0.77)	0.98 (0.82–1.17)	0.87 (0.72–1.06)	0.78 (0.61–1.00)	0.92 (0.77–1.10)	0.85 (0.78–0.93)

Points estimates are hazard ratio (95% confidence interval).

Abbreviations: 3P-MACE, three-point major adverse cardiovascular events (ie, a composite of myocardial infarction, stroke, or cardiovascular death); CANVAS, CANagliflozin cardioVascular Assessment Study; CREDENCE, canagliflozin and renal events in diabetes with established nephropathy clinical evaluation; CV, cardiovascular; DECLARE-TIMI 58, Dapagliflozin Effect on Cardiovascular Events–Thrombolysis in Myocardial Infarction 58; EMPA-REG OUTCOME, empagliflozin, Cardiovascular Outcomes, and Mortality in Type 2 Diabetes; HHF, hospitalization for heart failure; VERTIS-CV, eValuation of ERTugliflozin efficacy and Safety CardioVascular outcomes trial.

[a] McGuire DK, Shih WJ, Cosentino F, et al. Association of SGLT2 Inhibitors With Cardiovascular and Kidney Outcomes in Patients With Type 2 Diabetes: A Meta-analysis. *JAMA Cardiol.* Feb 1 2021;6(2):148-158. https://doi.org/10.1001/jamacardio.2020.4511.

In parallel, the Canagliflozin and Renal Events in Diabetes with Established Nephropathy Clinical Evaluation (CREDENCE) trial was conducted in patients with T2DM and chronic kidney disease: 4401 patients with T2DM with an estimated glomerular filtration rate ranging from 30 to 90 mL/min/1.73 m^2 were randomized to either canagliflozin or placebo on top of angiotensin-converting enzyme inhibitors.[30] The primary outcome was a composite of sustained (at least 30 days) doubling of serum creatinine, end-stage kidney disease, and death from renal or cardiovascular causes. The relative risk of the primary outcome was reduced by 30% in the canagliflozin group compared with placebo.[30] Patients who received canagliflozin also had a lower risk of cardiovascular death, myocardial infarction, or stroke (HR, 0.80; 95% CI, 0.67–0.95) and HHF (HR, 0.61; 95% CI, 0.47–0.80). Results of the CREDENCE trial were also examined by baseline hemoglobin A$_{1c}$ (HbA$_{1c}$), reporting that the benefit of canagliflozin on the primary outcome was consistent across HbA$_{1c}$ categories, even in those with levels lower than 7%, with no signals of increased serious adverse events.[31]

In the eValuation of ERTugliflozin efficacy and Safety CardioVascular outcomes trial (VERTIS-CV) trial, where 8246 patients with T2DM and ASCVD were randomized to ertugliflozin versus placebo, ertugliflozin was noninferior, but not superior, to placebo as regards the effect on 3P-MACE (HR, 0.97; 95.6% CI, 0.85–1.11) and on the time to first HHF/cardiovascular death (HR, 0.88; 95.8% CI, 0.75–1.03).[32] However, a prespecified analysis reported that ertugliflozin significantly reduced total HF-related events (ie, including first and recurrent events), by 30% and total HHF/cardiovascular death by 17%, regardless of presence of HF at baseline and of ejection fraction values.[33] Because VERTIS-CV included a higher proportion of patients with HF history at baseline (24%) compared with the other SGLT2i CVOTs, these results offered a particularly accurate insight of the total HF burden.[33]

Finally, a meta-analysis of pooled data from the reported CVOTs showed that SGLT2i reduce the risk of 3P-MACE by a modest 10% (HR, 0.90; 95% CI, 0.85–0.95), being demonstrated within trials for empagliflozin and canagliflozin only.[34] As regards cardiovascular death, the overall significant reduction offered by SGLT2i in patients with T2DM is of 15%, but only empagliflozin demonstrated significant outcomes for cardiovascular death risk reduction and the heterogeneity was 64%.[34] However, the most consistent effect of SGLT2i across trials was that on HHF, with a 32% relative risk reduction (HR, 0.68; 95% CI, 0.61–0.76) and no heterogeneity (**Fig. 1**).[34] There was no significant interaction between the use of SGLT2i and the presence of ASCVD and/or HF at baseline.[34]

More recently, efficacy and safety of the SGLT2/SGLT1i sotagliflozin was tested against placebo in the Sotagliflozin on Cardiovascular Events in Patients with Type 2 Diabetes Post Worsening Heart Failure (SOLOIST-WHF) trial, including 1222 patients with T2DM and a recent hospitalization for worsening HF.[35] Despite the trial being terminated early because of the COVID-19 pandemic, sotagliflozin significantly reduced the occurrence of the primary end point of HHF/urgent visits for HF and cardiovascular death (first and subsequent events) compared with placebo (51.0 vs 76.3 per 100 patient-years; HR, 0.67; 95% CI, 0.52–0.85).[35] Importantly, in SOLOIST, the first dose of the trial product was administered before hospital discharge or after a median of 2 days following discharge, supporting the safety of early initiation of SGLT2i in patients with HF.[35] The benefit of sotagliflozin was evident for all patients regardless of their ejection fraction, even though the small sample size of the subgroup with heart failure with preserved ejection fraction limits the finding on this subgroup.[35] Sotagliflozin was also tested in the Sotagliflozin on Cardiovascular and Renal Events in Patients with Type 2 Diabetes and Moderate Renal Impairment Who Are at Cardiovascular Risk (SCORED) trial, enrolling 10,540 patients with T2DM and chronic kidney disease (25–60 mL/min/1.73 m^2).[36] Sotagliflozin reduced the primary end point (ie, the composite of the total number of deaths from cardiovascular causes, HHF, and urgent HF visits) by 26% (HR, 0.74; 95% CI, 0.63–0.88); however, in the sotagliflozin group adverse events including diarrhea, genital mycotic infections, volume depletion, and diabetic ketoacidosis were more common.[36]

Taken together, these results paved the way for designing future trials to specifically assess the outcomes in patients with HF, regardless of the presence of T2DM.

THE SUPPORTING RESULTS FROM REAL-WORLD OBSERVATIONS

The first large observational study looking into the association between SGLT2i and HF outcomes in patients with T2DM was the Comparative Effectiveness of Cardiovascular Outcomes in New Users of SGLT-2 Inhibitors (CVD-REAL), collecting data from the United States, Sweden, Denmark, Norway, Germany, and the United Kingdom from 2012 to 2013. In this study, new users of empagliflozin, canagliflozin, and dapagliflozin were compared with other glucose-lowering drugs, for a total of 309,056 patients.[37] SGLT2i were associated with a lower risk of HHF (HR, 0.61; 95% CI, 0.51–0.73) and all-cause death (HR, 0.49; 95% CI, 0.41–0.57) compared with other antihyperglycemic medications.[37] The relative risks for HHF and death associated with SGLT2i use were similar in the two subgroups with and without established ASCVD, representing 13% and 87% of the study population, respectively.[38] However, the absolute event rates for HHF differed substantially, being higher in patients with established CVD at baseline (2.3/100 patient-years for SGLT2i users vs 3.2/100 patient-years for other glucose-lowering drugs) than in patients without established CVD (0.1/100 patient-years in those on SGLT2 inhibitors vs 0.9/100 patient-years for those on other glucose-lowering drugs).[38] This led to speculate that the number needed to treat in future randomized trials on HF outcomes in high-risk patients would be considerably lower in a patient population with established CVD at

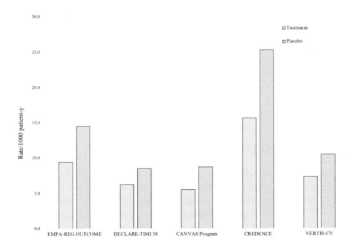

Fig. 1. Incidence rates of heart failure hospitalization in the treatment and placebo groups in each trial. CANVAS, CANagliflozin cardioVascular Assessment Study; CREDENCE, Canagliflozin and Renal Events in Diabetes with Established Nephropathy Clinical Evaluation; DECLARE-TIMI 58, Dapagliflozin Effect on Cardiovascular Events–Thrombolysis in Myocardial Infarction 58; EMPA-REG OUTCOME, Empagliflozin, Cardiovascular Outcomes, and Mortality in Type 2 Diabetes; VERTIS-CV, eValuation of ERTugliflozin effIcacy and Safety CardioVascular outcomes trial.

baseline, including history of HF; as mentioned, this was subsequently confirmed by the results of EMPA-REG OUTCOME. Moreover, the early divergence of the Kaplan-Meier curves for HHF and cardiovascular death in the previously mentioned CVOTs suggested a short duration of trials designated ad hoc for HF outcomes.

In EMPRISE, a large observational study conducted in the United States, empagliflozin was associated with a decreased risk of HHF by 50% (HR, 0.50; 95% CI, 0.28–0.91) compared with sitagliptin.[39] Accordingly, in a real-world meta-analysis of four observational databases from the United States canagliflozin therapy was associated with a lower risk of HHF compared with other glucose-lowering agents, with an HR of 0.39 (95% CI, 0.26–0.60).[39] SGLT2i use in patients with T2DM was associated with a 30% lower risk of first HHF and cardiovascular death in the Swedish HF registry, consistently across ejection fraction and renal function, in patients with and without baseline metformin treatment.[40]

FROM BEDSIDE TO BENCH: MECHANISMS OF ACTION OF SGLT2i

SGLT2i have a simple pharmacodynamic: by blocking sodium-glucose reabsorption in the proximal renal tubule of patients with T2DM, their use leads to increased renal glucose excretion and lower plasma glucose levels, and thus to HbA_{1c} and glucotoxicity reduction.[41–43] An overall improvement of the cardiovascular risk factor profile, including weight loss, fat mass reduction, lowering of blood pressure and arterial stiffness, and improvements in endothelial dysfunction, inflammation, and oxidative stress were initially studied.[44–48] As regards the hemodynamic effects induced by SGLT2i, the volume depletion does not activate the renin-angiotensin-aldosterone system or the sympathetic nervous system[49]; this is probably caused by the absence of change in intravascular volume, which is normally responsible for the deleterious neurohormonal activation.[49,50] As a result, SGLT2i likely exert a diuretic effect while also causing an efficient body fluid redistribution, reducing cardiac preload.[51]

Hemoconcentration emerged as a principal mechanism of the SGLT2i benefit from the EMPA-REG OUTCOME trial: the relative increase in hematocrit was 12% and changes in hematocrit and hemoglobin explained 52% and 49%, respectively, of the reduction of cardiovascular death seen with empagliflozin compared with placebo, reflecting the hemoconcentration and possibly a direct increase in erythropoietin secretion.[52–54] Similar evidence of hemoconcentration has been consistently observed in several SGLT2i trials.[49,55]

Diabetic cardiomyopathy is also counteracted by SGLT2 inhibition: myocardial metabolism is shifted from glucose and fatty acids use to ketones use, which is more energetically convenient.[53] In experimental models, SGLT2i attenuate myocardial hypertrophy, potentially by reducing pericoronary fibrosis, coronary arterial thickening, and cardiac macrophage infiltration.[56,57] This constituted the basis for the Effects of Empagliflozin on Cardiac Structure in Patients with Type 2 Diabetes (EMPA-HEART) study, where empagliflozin reduced left ventricular mass after 6 months in 97 patients with T2DM with coronary artery disease.[58]

However, the magnitude of such effects did not fully explain the striking results seen in HF trials: for example, in the trials in T2DM, the weight loss is of only 2 to 3 kg, and the blood pressure reduction is modest (systolic/diastolic: −3.6/-1.7 mm Hg).[52,59] Moreover, these were changes from baseline to the end of trials, but Kaplan-Meier curves for HHF-related outcomes diverged after only a few weeks. Therefore, after the positive results in HF trials, other mechanisms are being investigated. Altered sodium handling in cardiomyocytes is involved in HF progression[60] and the most important exchanger in sodium homeostasis, the sodium-nitrogen exchanger isoform 1 (NHE1), has an increased activity in HF.[61] Indeed, its abnormal activation induces hypertrophy and hyperactivity of the renin-angiotensin-aldosterone, sympathetic, and natriuretic peptide systems.[62] SGLT2i directly inhibit NHE1 in HF models with and without diabetes, counteracting this detrimental activation.[63–65] Moreover, this effect on cardiomyocyte ion homeostasis could be the mechanism underlying the association of SGLT2i treatment with reduced risk of arrhythmias, as suggested by a post hoc analysis of the DAPA-HF trial[66] and by a meta-analysis of SGLT2i trials in T2DM.[67] In addition, mitochondrial physiology is positively affected by normalization of sodium handling in the failing heart, restoring efficient energy supply, and reducing the formation of reactive oxygen species.[68,69] Further lines of research have been suggested, investigating the effect of SGLT1 inhibition and thus of nonselective SGLT1/SGLT2i.[70,71]

DISCLOSURE

The authors have no conflict of interest to disclose in relation to this present work. G.F. has received grant support from the Erling-Persson family foundation and from the Swedish Heart-Lung Foundation, Sweden; and speaker fees from the European Society of Cardiology, outside of the present work.

G.S. has received personal fees from Società Prodotti Antibiotici, Roche, Servier, GENESIS, Cytokinetics, and Medtronic; grants and personal fees from Vifor and AstraZeneca; grants and nonfinancial support from Boehringer-Ingelheim; and grants from Novartis, Boston Scientific, Bayer, United States, Merck, and Pharmacosmos outside the submitted work. F.C. reports personal fees from AstraZeneca, United Kingdom, Bayer, Germany, Boehringer-Ingelheim, Bristol-Myers Squibb, Merck Sharp & Dohme, Lilly, Novo Nordisk, and Pfizer; and grants from Swedish Research Council, Sweden, Swedish Heart-Lung Foundation, and the King Gustav V and Queen Victoria Foundation, outside the submitted work.

REFERENCES

1. Von Mrig J. Observations sur les proprietes febrifuges de la phloridzine. Bull Soc Med Gand 1836; 75–110.
2. von Mering J. Uber kunstlichen diabetes. Centralbl Med Wiss 1885;23:531–2.
3. Chasis H, Jolliffe N, Smith HW. The action of phlorizin on the excretion of glucose, xylose, sucrose, creatinine and urea by man. J Clin Invest 1933; 12(6):1083–90.
4. Alvarado F, Crane RK. Phlorizin as a competitive inhibitor of the active transport of sugars by hamster small intestine, in vitro. Biochim Biophys Acta 1962;56:170–2.
5. Vick H, Diedrich DF, Baumann K. Reevaluation of renal tubular glucose transport inhibition by phlorizin analogs. Am J Physiol 1973;224(3):552–7.
6. Shepherd PR, Kahn BB. Glucose transporters and insulin action: implications for insulin resistance and diabetes mellitus. N Engl J Med 1999;341(4):248–57.
7. Wood IS, Trayhurn P. Glucose transporters (GLUT and SGLT): expanded families of sugar transport proteins. Br J Nutr 2003;89(1):3–9.
8. Ehrenkranz JR, Lewis NG, Kahn CR, Roth J. Phlorizin: a review. Diabetes Metab Res Rev 2005;21(1): 31–8.
9. Oku A, Ueta K, Arakawa K, et al. T-1095, an inhibitor of renal Na+-glucose cotransporters, may provide a novel approach to treating diabetes. Diabetes 1999; 48(9):1794–800.
10. Ueta K, Ishihara T, Matsumoto Y, et al. Long-term treatment with the Na+-glucose cotransporter inhibitor T-1095 causes sustained improvement in hyperglycemia and prevents diabetic neuropathy in Goto-Kakizaki Rats. Life Sci 2005;76(23):2655–68.
11. Ferrannini G, Savarese G, Ryden L. Sodium-glucose transporter inhibition in heart failure: from an unexpected side effect to a novel treatment possibility. Diabetes Res Clin Pract 2021;175:108796.
12. Nissen SE, Wolski K. Effect of rosiglitazone on the risk of myocardial infarction and death from cardiovascular causes. N Engl J Med 2007;356(24): 2457–71.
13. Hennekens CH, Hebert PR, Schneider WR, O'Brien P, Demets D, Borer JS. Academic perspectives on the United States Food and Drug Administration's guidance for industry on diabetes mellitus. Contemp Clin Trials 2010;31(5):411–3.
14. Zinman B, Wanner C, Lachin JM, et al. Empagliflozin, cardiovascular outcomes, and mortality in type 2 diabetes. N Engl J Med 2015;373(22):2117–28.
15. Fitchett D, Zinman B, Wanner C, et al. Heart failure outcomes with empagliflozin in patients with type 2 diabetes at high cardiovascular risk: results of the EMPA-REG OUTCOME(R) trial. Eur Heart J 2016; 37(19):1526–34.
16. Fitchett D, Butler J, van de Borne P, et al. Effects of empagliflozin on risk for cardiovascular death and heart failure hospitalization across the spectrum of heart failure risk in the EMPA-REG OUTCOME(R) trial. Eur Heart J 2018;39(5):363–70.
17. Savarese G, Sattar N, Januzzi J, et al. Empagliflozin is associated with a lower risk of post-acute heart failure rehospitalization and mortality. Circulation 2019;139(11):1458–60.
18. Zannad F, McMurray JJ, Krum H, et al. Eplerenone in patients with systolic heart failure and mild symptoms. N Engl J Med 2011;364(1):11–21.
19. Effects of enalapril on mortality in severe congestive heart failure. Results of the Cooperative North Scandinavian Enalapril Survival Study (CONSENSUS). N Engl J Med 1987;316(23):1429–35.
20. Wiviott SD, Raz I, Bonaca MP, et al. Dapagliflozin and cardiovascular outcomes in type 2 diabetes. N Engl J Med 2019;380(4):347–57.
21. Furtado RHM, Bonaca MP, Raz I, et al. Dapagliflozin and cardiovascular outcomes in patients with type 2 diabetes mellitus and previous myocardial infarction. Circulation 2019;139(22):2516–27.
22. Zelniker TA, Morrow DA, Mosenzon O, et al. Relationship between baseline cardiac biomarkers and cardiovascular death or hospitalization for heart failure with and without sodium-glucose co-transporter 2 inhibitor therapy in DECLARE-TIMI 58. Eur J Heart Fail 2020. https://doi.org/10.1002/ejhf.2073.
23. Bajaj HS, Raz I, Mosenzon O, et al. Cardiovascular and renal benefits of dapagliflozin in patients with short and long-standing type 2 diabetes: analysis from the DECLARE-TIMI 58 trial. Diabetes Obes Metab 2020;22(7):1122–31.
24. Kato ET, Silverman MG, Mosenzon O, et al. Effect of dapagliflozin on heart failure and mortality in type 2 diabetes mellitus. Circulation 2019;139(22):2528–36.
25. Neal B, Perkovic V, Mahaffey KW, et al. Canagliflozin and cardiovascular and renal events in type 2 diabetes. N Engl J Med 2017;377(7):644–57.

26. Mahaffey KW, Jardine MJ, Bompoint S, et al. Canagliflozin and cardiovascular and renal outcomes in type 2 diabetes mellitus and chronic kidney disease in primary and secondary cardiovascular prevention groups. Circulation 2019;140(9):739–50.

27. Radholm K, Figtree G, Perkovic V, et al. Canagliflozin and heart failure in type 2 diabetes mellitus: results from the CANVAS Program. Circulation 2018; 138(5):458–68.

28. Ohkuma T, Van Gaal L, Shaw W, et al. Clinical outcomes with canagliflozin according to baseline body mass index: results from post hoc analyses of the CANVAS Program. Diabetes Obes Metab 2020;22(4):530–9.

29. Neuen BL, Ohkuma T, Neal B, et al. Cardiovascular and renal outcomes with canagliflozin according to baseline kidney function. Circulation 2018;138(15): 1537–50.

30. Perkovic V, Jardine MJ, Neal B, et al. Canagliflozin and renal outcomes in type 2 diabetes and nephropathy. N Engl J Med 2019;380(24):2295–306.

31. Cannon CP, Perkovic V, Agarwal R, et al. Evaluating the effects of canagliflozin on cardiovascular and renal events in patients with type 2 diabetes mellitus and chronic kidney disease according to baseline HbA1c, including those with HbA1c <7%: results from the CREDENCE Trial. Circulation 2020;141(5): 407–10. https://doi.org/10.1161/circulationaha.119. 044359.

32. Cannon CP, Pratley R, Dagogo-Jack S, et al. Cardiovascular outcomes with ertugliflozin in type 2 diabetes. N Engl J Med 2020;383(15):1425–35.

33. Cosentino F, Cannon CP, Cherney DZI, et al. Efficacy of ertugliflozin on heart failure-related events in patients with type 2 diabetes mellitus and established atherosclerotic cardiovascular disease: results of the VERTIS CV Trial. Circulation 2020;142(23): 2205–15.

34. McGuire DK, Shih WJ, Cosentino F, et al. Association of SGLT2 inhibitors with cardiovascular and kidney outcomes in patients with type 2 diabetes: a meta-analysis. JAMA Cardiol 2021;6(2):148–58.

35. Bhatt DL, Szarek M, Steg PG, et al. Sotagliflozin in patients with diabetes and recent worsening heart failure. N Engl J Med 2021;384(2):117–28. https:// doi.org/10.1056/NEJMoa2030183.

36. Bhatt DL, Szarek M, Pitt B, et al. Sotagliflozin in patients with diabetes and chronic kidney disease. N Engl J Med 2020;16. https://doi.org/10.1056/ NEJMoa2030186.

37. Kosiborod M, Cavender MA, Fu AZ, et al. Lower risk of heart failure and death in patients initiated on sodium-glucose cotransporter-2 inhibitors versus other glucose-lowering drugs: the CVD-REAL Study (Comparative Effectiveness of Cardiovascular Outcomes in New Users of Sodium-Glucose Cotransporter-2 Inhibitors). Circulation 2017;136(3):249–59.

38. Cavender MA, Norhammar A, Birkeland KI, et al. SGLT-2 inhibitors and cardiovascular risk: an analysis of CVD-REAL. J Am Coll Cardiol 2018;71(22): 2497–506.

39. Ryan PB, Buse JB, Schuemie MJ, et al. Comparative effectiveness of canagliflozin, SGLT2 inhibitors and non-SGLT2 inhibitors on the risk of hospitalization for heart failure and amputation in patients with type 2 diabetes mellitus: a real-world meta-analysis of 4 observational databases (OBSERVE-4D). Diabetes Obes Metab 2018;20(11):2585–97.

40. Becher PM, Schrage B, Ferrannini G, et al. Use of sodium-glucose co-transporter 2 inhibitors in patients with heart failure and type 2 diabetes mellitus: data from the Swedish Heart Failure Registry. Eur J Heart Fail 2021. https://doi.org/10.1002/ejhf.2131.

41. Scheen AJ. Cardiovascular effects of new oral glucose-lowering agents: DPP-4 and SGLT-2 inhibitors. Circ Res 2018;122(10):1439–59.

42. Monami M, Liistro F, Scatena A, Nreu B, Mannucci E. Short and medium-term efficacy of sodium glucose co-transporter-2 (SGLT-2) inhibitors: a meta-analysis of randomized clinical trials. Diabetes Obes Metab 2018;20(5):1213–22.

43. Cowie MR, Fisher M. SGLT2 inhibitors: mechanisms of cardiovascular benefit beyond glycaemic control. Nat Rev Cardiol 2020;17(12):761–72.

44. Ferrannini G, Rydén L. Sodium-glucose transporter 2 inhibition and cardiovascular events in patients with diabetes: information from clinical trials and observational real-world data. Clin Sci (Lond) 2018;132(18):2003–12.

45. Ferrannini E, Solini A. SGLT2 inhibition in diabetes mellitus: rationale and clinical prospects. Nat Rev Endocrinol 2012;8(8):495–502.

46. Heerspink HJ, Perkins BA, Fitchett DH, Husain M, Cherney DZ. Sodium glucose cotransporter 2 inhibitors in the treatment of diabetes mellitus: cardiovascular and kidney effects, potential mechanisms, and clinical applications. Circulation 2016;134(10): 752–72.

47. Ridderstråle M, Andersen KR, Zeller C, Kim G, Woerle HJ, Broedl UC. Comparison of empagliflozin and glimepiride as add-on to metformin in patients with type 2 diabetes: a 104-week randomised, active-controlled, double-blind, phase 3 trial. Lancet Diabetes Endocrinol 2014;2(9):691–700.

48. Baker WL, Smyth LR, Riche DM, Bourret EM, Chamberlin KW, White WB. Effects of sodium-glucose co-transporter 2 inhibitors on blood pressure: a systematic review and meta-analysis. J Am Soc Hypertens 2014;8(4):262–75.e9.

49. Griffin M, Rao VS, Ivey-Miranda J, et al. Empagliflozin in heart failure: diuretic and cardiorenal effects. Circulation 2020;142(11):1028–39.

50. Jensen J, Omar M, Kistorp C, et al. Effects of empagliflozin on estimated extracellular volume,

estimated plasma volume, and measured glomerular filtration rate in patients with heart failure (Empire HF Renal): a prespecified substudy of a double-blind, randomised, placebo-controlled trial. Lancet Diabetes Endocrinol 2021;9(2):106–16.

51. Verma S, McMurray JJV. SGLT2 inhibitors and mechanisms of cardiovascular benefit: a state-of-the-art review. Diabetologia 2018;61(10):2108–17.

52. Inzucchi SE, Zinman B, Wanner C, et al. SGLT-2 inhibitors and cardiovascular risk: proposed pathways and review of ongoing outcome trials. Diab Vasc Dis Res 2015;12(2):90–100.

53. Ferrannini E, Baldi S, Frascerra S, et al. Shift to fatty substrate utilization in response to sodium-glucose cotransporter 2 inhibition in subjects without diabetes and patients with type 2 diabetes. Diabetes 2016;65(5):1190–5.

54. Inzucchi SE, Zinman B, Fitchett D, et al. How does empagliflozin reduce cardiovascular mortality? Insights from a mediation analysis of the EMPA-REG OUTCOME Trial. Diabetes Care 2018;41(2):356–63.

55. Sha S, Polidori D, Heise T, et al. Effect of the sodium glucose co-transporter 2 inhibitor canagliflozin on plasma volume in patients with type 2 diabetes mellitus. Diabetes Obes Metab 2014;16(11):1087–95.

56. Lin B, Koibuchi N, Hasegawa Y, et al. Glycemic control with empagliflozin, a novel selective SGLT2 inhibitor, ameliorates cardiovascular injury and cognitive dysfunction in obese and type 2 diabetic mice. Cardiovasc Diabetol 2014;13:148.

57. Lee TM, Chang NC, Lin SZ. Dapagliflozin, a selective SGLT2 inhibitor, attenuated cardiac fibrosis by regulating the macrophage polarization via STAT3 signaling in infarcted rat hearts. Free Radic Biol Med 2017;104:298–310.

58. Verma S, Mazer CD, Yan AT, et al. Effect of empagliflozin on left ventricular mass in patients with type 2 diabetes mellitus and coronary artery disease: the EMPA-HEART CardioLink-6 randomized clinical trial. Circulation 2019;140(21):1693–702.

59. Georgianos PI, Agarwal R. Ambulatory blood pressure reduction with SGLT-2 inhibitors: dose-response meta-analysis and comparative evaluation with low-dose hydrochlorothiazide. Diabetes Care 2019;42(4):693–700.

60. Weber CR, Piacentino V 3rd, Houser SR, Bers DM. Dynamic regulation of sodium/calcium exchange function in human heart failure. Circulation 2003;108(18):2224–9.

61. Yokoyama H, Gunasegaram S, Harding SE, Avkiran M. Sarcolemmal Na+/H+ exchanger activity and expression in human ventricular myocardium. J Am Coll Cardiol 2000;36(2):534–40.

62. Padan E, Landau M. Sodium-proton (Na(+)/H(+)) antiporters: properties and roles in health and disease. Met Ions Life Sci 2016;16:391–458.

63. Trum M, Riechel J, Lebek S, et al. Empagliflozin inhibits Na(+)/H(+) exchanger activity in human atrial cardiomyocytes. ESC Heart Fail 2020. https://doi.org/10.1002/ehf2.13024.

64. Yurista SR, Sillje HHW, Oberdorf-Maass SU, et al. Sodium-glucose co-transporter 2 inhibition with empagliflozin improves cardiac function in non-diabetic rats with left ventricular dysfunction after myocardial infarction. Eur J Heart Fail 2019;21(7):862–73.

65. Cappetta D, De Angelis A, Ciuffreda LP, et al. Amelioration of diastolic dysfunction by dapagliflozin in a non-diabetic model involves coronary endothelium. Pharmacol Res Jul 2020;157:104781.

66. Curtain JP, Docherty KF, Jhund PS, et al. Effect of dapagliflozin on ventricular arrhythmias, resuscitated cardiac arrest, or sudden death in DAPA-HF. Eur Heart J 2021;42(36):3727–38.

67. Fernandes GC, Fernandes A, Cardoso R, et al. Association of SGLT2 inhibitors with arrhythmias and sudden cardiac death in patients with type 2 diabetes or heart failure: a meta-analysis of 34 randomized controlled trials. Heart Rhythm 2021;18(7):1098–105.

68. Liu T, O'Rourke B. Enhancing mitochondrial Ca2+ uptake in myocytes from failing hearts restores energy supply and demand matching. Circ Res 2008;103(3):279–88.

69. Baartscheer A, Schumacher CA, Wust RC, et al. Empagliflozin decreases myocardial cytoplasmic Na(+) through inhibition of the cardiac Na(+)/H(+) exchanger in rats and rabbits. Diabetologia 2017;60(3):568–73.

70. Young SL, Ryan L, Mullins TP, et al. Sotagliflozin, a dual SGLT1/2 inhibitor, improves cardiac outcomes in a normoglycemic mouse model of cardiac pressure overload. Front Physiol 2021;12:738594.

71. Pitt B, Bhatt DL. Does SGLT1 inhibition add benefit to SGLT2 inhibition in type 2 diabetes? Circulation 2021;144(1):4–6.

SGLT2 Inhibitors in Heart Failure with Reduced Ejection Fraction

A Paradigm Shift Toward Dual Cardio-Renal Protection

Tripti Rastogi, MD, MSc, Nicolas Girerd, MD, PhD*

KEYWORDS

- SGLT2i • HFrEF • Cardiovascular outcomes • Renal outcomes

KEY POINTS

- Sodium-glucose cotransporter-2 inhibitors (SGLT2i) substantially improve cardiovascular and renal outcomes in heart failure with reduced ejection fraction (HFrEF).
- Midterm renoprotective effects of SGLT2i may facilitate the continuation of recommended doses of angiotensin converting enzyme inhibitors or neprilysin inhibitor and mineralocorticoid antagonists.
- Current evidence suggests a likely benefit in initiating all HFrEF drugs concomitantly (or within a very-short timeframe) at low dose and subsequently up-titrate.

BACKGROUND

Heart failure (HF) remains one of the leading causes of morbidity and mortality worldwide. Despite considerable advances in therapy, prognosis remains poor in heart failure with reduced ejection fraction (HFrEF). Current guidelines recommend foundational therapy consisting of angiotensin converting enzyme inhibitors (ACEi)/angiotensin-neprilysin inhibitor (ARNi), mineralocorticoid antagonists (MRAs) and ß-blockers to prevent adverse outcomes. Recently, sodium-glucose cotransporter-2 inhibitors (SGLT2i) have been approved for the treatment and prevention of HFrEF in conjunction with foundational therapy.[1,2]

Cardiovascular, metabolic, and renal diseases are interlinked with one another due to the commonality of risk factors. HF and chronic kidney disease (CKD) can moreover be regarded as a cardiorenal continuum given that they share several common risk factors and disease pathways that interact with each other,[3] such that the presence of one worsens the prognosis of the other and vice versa.

Originally developed for the treatment of type 2 diabetes, SGLT2i lower the risk of both cardiovascular and renal outcomes in patients with HFrEF, CKD, and/or at high risk of HF.[4–8] In the present article, we review the cardiovascular and renal benefits of SGLT2i in HFrEF, as well as their preventive potential against progression to HF.

EVIDENCE OF THE BENEFITS OF SODIUM-GLUCOSE COTRANSPORTER-2 INHIBITORS ON CARDIOVASCULAR OUTCOMES IN PATIENTS WITH HEART FAILURE WITH REDUCED EJECTION FRACTION

Cardiovascular outcome trials performed in type 2 diabetes indicated that SGLT2i prevent adverse cardiovascular outcomes in patients with diabetes and high cardiovascular risk.[7–9] These findings generated the hypothesis that SGLT2i may have similar beneficial effects in HFrEF irrespective of diabetes status.

Centre d'Investigation Clinique Pierre Drouin -INSERM - CHRU de Nancy, Institut lorrain du cœur et des vaisseaux Louis Mathieu, Nancy, France
* Corresponding author. 4, rue du Morvan, Vandœuvre-Lès-Nancy 54500.
E-mail address: nicolas_girerd@yahoo.com

Heart Failure Clin 18 (2022) 561–577
https://doi.org/10.1016/j.hfc.2022.03.006
1551-7136/22/© 2022 Elsevier Inc. All rights reserved.

heartfailure.theclinics.com

Sodium-glucose cotransporter-2 inhibitors in Chronic Stable Heart Failure with Reduced Ejection Fraction

Two large pivotal clinical trials, DAPA-HF and EMPEROR-Reduced, provided convincing evidence that SGLT2i reduce adverse cardiovascular outcomes in HFrEF.[4,5] Based on these results, SGLT2i were approved as the initial treatment in HFrEF, in combination with foundational therapy.

Both DAPA-HF and EMPEROR-Reduced trials included patients with chronic stable HFrEF irrespective of diabetes status—and eventually included approximately 50% of patients with diabetes (**Table 1**). DAPA-HF was conducted in relatively low-risk patients, whereas the EMPEROR-Reduced trial used risk-enrichment strategies by enrolling patients with markedly reduced left ventricular ejection fraction (LVEF) or patients with reduced LVEF (30%–40%) with increased levels of N-terminal pro-brain natriuretic peptide (NT-pro-BNP) (depending on the range of LVEF and heart rhythm). Given these differences in inclusion criteria, these 2 trials investigated the effects of SGLT2i over a wide range of disease states and risk factors. Patients were approximately 65 years old and one-fifth of the trial population in both trials were women. In EMPEROR-Reduced, mean LVEF (27%) and glomerular filtration rate (eGFR) (62 mL/min/1.73 m^2) were numerically lower compared with DAPA-HF (mean LVEF 31% and eGFR 66 mL/min/1.73 m^2). The primary composite outcome was similar in both trials and consisted of cardiovascular mortality and hospitalization for HF. In DAPA-HF, the primary composite outcome also included an urgent visit resulting in intravenous therapy for HF as a component of primary outcome, which has been shown to be strongly associated with subsequent outcome.[4] This latter component of the composite outcome is likely to become standard with the emergence of ambulatory approaches for managing worsening HF.

In both trials, the primary outcome was significantly reduced and the magnitude of effect was in fact nearly identical (DAPA-HF: 0.74 [0.65–0.85], EMPEROR-Reduced: 0.75 [0.65–0.86]) (Figure: **Fig. 2** Graphical Abstract). In DAPA-HF, all components of the primary composite outcome were significantly reduced. However, in EMPEROR-Reduced, the reduction in primary outcome was driven by a reduction in hospitalization for HF. This difference was perhaps due to differences in participants' baseline characteristics or trial duration.[10] Statistical power issues may also be at play because EMPEROR-Reduced had a smaller sample size (n = 3730 vs 4744) and a shorter follow-up (16 vs 18.2 months) compared with DAPA-HF. A meta-analysis of the 2 trials using pooled study-level data (DAPA-HF) and patient-level data (EMPEROR-Reduced) showed that SGLT2i reduced all-cause mortality by 13% in patients with different clinical profiles, without significant evidence of heterogeneity across the trials.[11]

Sodium-glucose cotransporter-2 inhibitors in acute heart failure

A pilot randomized controlled trial (EMPA-RESPONSE-AHF) explored the effects of empagliflozin on symptoms, diuretic response, and change in NT-pro-BNP level from baseline to day 4 and on the combined endpoint of in-hospital worsening of HF, all-cause mortality and/or HF readmission at day 60 in patients with acute HF (n = 80).[12] Empagliflozin increased urinary output during the initial 4 days of treatment and significantly reduced the combined endpoints compared with placebo during 60 days.

In the SOLOIST-WHF trial, the effects of SGLT2i were studied irrespective of LVEF (although median LVEF was eventually 35%) in worsening HF.[13] Sotagliflozin was associated with a lower total number of deaths from cardiovascular causes, hospitalizations and urgent visits for HF compared with placebo (hazard ratio [HR]: 0.67 [0.52–0.85]). During a median follow-up of 9 months, sotagliflozin reduced cardiovascular death and first hospitalization for worsening HF by 29% (HR: 0.71 [0.56–0.89]). The HRs in SOLOIST-WHF were almost identical to the results of clinical trials in chronic stable HFrEF.

In the EMPULSE trial, the effect of early initiation of SGLT2i in acute HF was assessed using a Win-ratio approach. Four events were hierarchically considered: death, number of HF events (eg, hospitalizations for HF, urgent HF visits, and unplanned outpatient visits), time to first HF event, and change from baseline in Kansas City Cardiomyopathy Questionnaire—Total Symptom Score (KCCQ-TSS).[14] Empagliflozin was associated with a significant improvement in the above conditions (win ratio 1.36 [1.09–1.68], P = .0054). Of note, empagliflozin was associated with fewer deaths compared with placebo (4.2% vs 8.3%).[14] Considering together, the results of the 3 aforementioned trials suggest that an early initiation of SGLT2i in hospitalized patients with acute HF can sizably reduce subsequent hospitalization and mortality.

Sodium-glucose cotransporter-2 inhibitors in heart failure with reduced ejection fraction according to comorbidities

The numerous, post hoc and subgroup analyses of the DAPA-HF and EMPEROR-Reduced trials reported that SGLT2i were associated with similar risk reductions in patients with HFrEF irrespective

Table 1
Cardiovascular and renal outcomes in pivotal trials and subgroup analyses of SGLT2i in HFrEF[a]

Trial Name	Patient Population and Subgroups in Post hoc Trials	Objective	Primary Endpoint	Results	Author, Year
DAPA-HF Duration: 18.2 mo N = 4744	**HFrEF with or without diabetes**	**To assess the efficacy and safety of the SGLT2 inhibitor dapagliflozin in patients with HFrEF**	**The primary CV outcome: a composite of WHF (hospitalization or an urgent visit resulting in IV therapy for HF) or CV death**	**HR: 0.74 (0.65–0.85)**	McMurray et al,[4] 2019
			Renal composite outcome	**HR: 0.71 (0.44–1.16)**	
	Patients with ischemic and nonischemic etiology	Efficacy according to ischemic and nonischemic etiology	The primary CV outcome	Patients with ischemia: HR 0.77, (0.65–0.92), Patients without ischemia HR 0.71, (0.58–0.87), P-interaction = 0.55)	Butt et al,[15] 2021
	Duration since the diagnosis of HF	Efficacy in relation to time from the diagnosis of HF	The primary CV outcome	≥2 to ≤12 mo: HR: 0.86 (0.63–1.18), >1–2 y: HR: 0.95 (0.64–1.42), >2–5 y: HR: 0.74 (0.57–0.96), >5 y: HR: 0.64 (0.53–0.78) P-interaction = 0.26	Yeoh et al,[21] 2020
	Patients with and without COPD	Outcomes related to COPD	The primary CV outcome	Patients with COPD: HR 0.67 (0.48–0.93) Without COPD: HR 0.76 (0.65–0.87); P-interaction = 0.47	Dewan et al,[19] 2021
	Age group of participants: <55, 55–64, 65–74, ≥75 y	The efficacy and safety of therapies in the elderly	The primary CV outcome	<55: HR: 0.87 (0.60–1.28), 55–64: HR: 0.71 (0.55–0.93), 65–74: HR: 0.76 (0.61–0.95), ≥75 y: HR: 0.68 (0.53–0.88). P-interaction: = 0.76	Martinez et al,[20] 2020

(continued on next page)

Table 1
(continued)

Trial Name	Patient Population and Subgroups in Post hoc Trials	Objective	Primary Endpoint	Results	Author, Year
	KCCQ-TSS score tertiles ≤65.6, 65.7–87.5, ≥87.5	The effects of dapagliflozin on a broad range of health status outcomes KCCQ	The primary CV outcome	KCCQ-TSS tertiles <65.6: HR: 0.70 (0.57–0.86); 65.7–87.5: HR: 0.77 (0.61–0.98), ≥87.5: HR: 0.62 (0.46–0.83)	Kosiborod,[36] 2020
	Treated with or without ARNi at baseline	Efficacy of dapagliflozin in patients depending on sacubitril/valsartan use at baseline	The primary CV outcome	Taking ARNi HR: 0.75(0.50–1.13) Not taking ARNi HR: 0.74 (0.65–0.86)	Solomon et al,[26] 2020
	With and without diabetes	Assess the effects of dapagliflozin in patients with HFrEF with and without diabetes	The primary CV outcome	With diabetes HR: 0.75 (0.63–0.90) Without diabetes HR: 0.73 (0.60–0.88) P-interaction: 0.8	Petrie et al,[22] 2020
EMPEROR-Reduced Duration = 16 mo N = 3730	**Preferential enrollment of patients with HFrEF with a greater severity of LVSD.**	**The effects of empagliflozin in patients across the broad spectrum of HFrEF**	**The primary outcome was a composite of CV death or HHF, analyzed as the time to first event.** Renal composite outcome	**HR: 0.75(0.65–0.86)** HR: 0.50 (0.32–0.77)	Packer et al,[5] 2020
	Patients receiving and not receiving ARNi	Influence of ARNi on the efficacy and safety of empagliflozin	Primary outcome	Patients receiving ARNi: HR: 0.64 (0.45–0.89) Patients not receiving ARNi: HR: 0.77 (0.66–0.90), P = .0008, interaction P = .31	Packer et al,[23] 2021
	Patients receiving and not receiving MRAs	To study the mutual influence of empagliflozin and MRAs in EMPEROR-Reduced	Primary outcome	In MRA nonusers: empagliflozin vs placebo: 0.76 (0.59–0.97); Receiving an MRA: empagliflozin vs placebo: 0.75 (0.63–	Ferreira et al,[25] 2021

	KCCQ-CSS tertiles at 3, 8, and 12 mo	Assess whether the benefits of empagliflozin varied by baseline health status and impact of empagliflozin on patient-reported outcomes	Primary outcome	0.88) (p-interaction: 0.93). KCCQ-CSS tertiles <62.5: HR: 0.83 (0.68–1.02); 62.6–85.4: HR: 0.74 (0.58–0.94), ≥85.4: HR: 0.61 (0.46–0.82) P-trend = 0.10	Butler et al,[35] 2021
	Groups according to SBP at baseline (<110; 110–130; >130 mm Hg)	Assess the interplay of SBP and the effects of empagliflozin	Primary outcome	SBP >130: HR: 0.82 (0.62–1.09); 110–130: HR: 0.71 (0.58–0.87); <110: HR: 0.78 (0.61–1.00)	Bohm, 2021[55]
SOLOIST-WHF Duration = 9 mo N = 1222 (EF<50% = 966)	Patients with type 2 DM and AHF	Safety and efficacy of SGLT2i when initiated soon after an acute HF episode	Total number of deaths from CV causes and hospitalizations and urgent visits for heart failure (first and subsequent events)	HR: 0.67 (0.52–0.85)	Bhatt et al,[13] 2021
EMPA-RESPONSE-AHF N = 80	AHF	Safety and clinical efficacy of SGLT2i in patients with AHF	Change in VAS dyspnea score: Diuretic response at day 4 Length of stay Percentage change in NT-pro-BNP at day 4	No difference was observed in VAS dyspnea score, diuretic response, length of stay, or change in NT-pro-BNP between empagliflozin and placebo	Damman et al,[12] 2020
EMPULSE-HF Duration = 90 d N = 530	Patients hospitalized for acute HF		Composite of death. Number of HF events, urgent/unplanned visits using Win-ratio approach	HR: 1.36 (1.09–1.68), P = .0054	Bavry et al,14 2021

(continued on next page)

Table 1
(continued)

Trial Name	Patient Population and Subgroups in Post hoc Trials	Objective	Primary Endpoint	Results	Author, Year
EMPIRE-HF Duration = 12 wk N = 190	Patients with HFrEF	**To investigate the effect of empagliflozin on NT-pro-BNP in HFrEF**	**Primary endpoint was the between-group difference in the change of NT-pro-BNP from baseline to 12 wk**	**Adjusted ratio of change empagliflozin/ placebo 0.98 (0.82– 1.11)**	Jensen et al,[39] 2020
Empire-HF renal Duration = 12 wk N = 120	Patients with HFrEF	To investigate the effects of empagliflozin on estimated extracellular volume, estimated plasma volume, measured GFR	The between-group difference in the changes in estimated extracellular volume, estimated plasma volume, and measured GFR from baseline to 12 wk	Empagliflozin resulted in reductions in estimated extracellular volume (−0·12 L (−0·18 to −0·05); P = 0·00,056), estimated plasma volume (−7·3%, −10·3 to −4·3; P < 0·0001), and measured GFR (−7·5 mL/min, −11·2 to −3·8; P = 0·00,010)	Jensen et al,[29] 2021

Abbreviation: AHF, acute heart failure; ARNi, angiotensin receptor/neprilysin inhibitor; COPD, chronic obstructive pulmonary disease; CV, cardiovascular; DM, diabetes mellitus; HF, heart failure; HR, hazard ratio; KCCQ, Kansas City Cardiomyopathy Questionnaire; MRA, mineralocorticoid receptor antagonists; OR, odds ratio; SBP, systolic blood pressure; VAS, visual analog scale.

[a] First line in bold presents the results of the primary outcome in the trial and subsequent lines present the results of secondary analyses.

of older age, cause and duration of HF, or the presence of chronic obstructive pulmonary disease, diabetes and impaired renal function (details in **Table 1**).[15–22] Overall, no sizable differences in the treatment response have been identified.

Sodium-glucose cotransporter-2 inhibitors in heart failure with reduced ejection fraction according to background medication

SGLT2i are well-tolerated in the presence of background therapy (diuretics, ACEi/ARNi, ß-blockers, and MRAs) and reduce the risk of adverse cardiovascular outcome irrespective of background therapy.[23–26]

Coadministration of ARNi with SGLT2i may have additional benefits over the treatment with ARNi due to their differing mechanisms in HFrEF.[23,27] Aside from this pharmacologic reasoning, the pooled subgroup analysis of the DAPA-HF and EMPEROR-Reduced trials showed that SGLT2i are equally effective in reducing hospitalization for HF and cardiovascular mortality irrespective of background ARNi treatment.[11] Similarly, SGLT2i were equally effective in MRA users and nonusers (HR: 0.75 [0.63–0.88] and 0.76 [0.59–0.97], respectively) in EMPEROR-Reduced.[25]

SGLT2i may furthermore facilitate the use of other HF drugs. A secondary analysis of EMPEROR-Reduced showed that SGLT2i were associated with lower rates of discontinuation of MRAs [0.78 (0.64–0.96)] in MRA users during follow-up.[25] In this analysis, empagliflozin was also associated with a lower risk of severe hyperkalemia (>6 mmol/L; HR: 0.70 [0.47–1.04]). Overall, the lower risk of hyperkalemia and fewer MRA discontinuations in patients treated with empagliflozin underscore that SGLT2i may favor MRA use.

Evidence of Sodium-Glucose cotransporter-2 Inhibitors Benefit on Renal Outcomes in Patients with Heart Failure with Reduced Ejection Fraction

Much of the evidence on the efficacy of SGLT2i on renal outcomes in HFrEF is based on the subsequent analyses of the prespecified secondary outcomes in the DAPA-HF and EMPEROR-Reduced trials. Approximately half of the patients enrolled in DAPA-HF and EMPEROR-Reduced had CKD (41% and 48%, respectively). Of note, renal outcomes were defined slightly differently in the 2 trials. In DAPA-HF, the composite renal outcome was defined as 50% or greater sustained decline in eGFR, end-stage kidney disease, and renal death. In EMPEROR-Reduced, the composite renal outcome was rather defined as time to first occurrence of chronic dialysis, kidney transplant, sustained reduction of 40% or greater eGFR, or

sustained eGFR less than 15 mL/min/1.73 m^2 if eGFR was greater than 30 mL/min/1.73 m^2 or less than 10 mL/min/1.73 m^2 for patients with baseline eGFR ≤30 mL/min/1.73 m^2.

The secondary analyses of both trials assessed the benefits of dapagliflozin and empagliflozin depending on the baseline renal function and whether dapagliflozin and empagliflozin had an effect on renal function.[18,28] In DAPA-HF, dapagliflozin was not associated with a significant reduction in composite renal outcome (HR = 0.71 [0.44–1.16], P = .17),[4,28] whereas empagliflozin significantly reduced composite renal outcome (HR = 0.50 [0.32–0.77]).[5] The favorable effects of empagliflozin remained similar even when the definition of CKD in DAPA-HF was applied in EMPEROR-Reduced.[11] The lack of significant association of dapagliflozin with renal outcomes in DAPA-HF is likely due to lower statistical power because patients included in DAPA-HF were at a relatively lower risk of outcome at baseline. It should be emphasized that the association of SGLT2i with renal outcomes, even if not significant, seemed sizable in DAPA-HF (HR = 0.71, ie, 29% reduction in renal outcomes) and that the association of dapagliflozin with eGFR slope, a more insightful outcome in a relatively low risk population, was significant (see below). In fact, when the treatment effects of the 2 trials were assessed in the meta-analysis, SGLT2i were associated with a significant reduction in primary renal outcome (using the DAPA-HF definition; HR: 0.62 [0.43–0.90]) with no significant heterogeneity.[11]

It should also be emphasized that both dapagliflozin and empagliflozin reduced the slope of eGFR decline in a very homogenous manner in patients with HFrEF. Dapagliflozin significantly reduced the rate of decline in eGFR between day 14 and 720: −1.09 (−1.40 to −0.77) versus placebo −2.85 (−3.17 to −2.53) mL/min/1.73 m^2/year.[28] Similarly, empagliflozin was associated with a slower annual rate of eGFR decline compared with the placebo group (−0.55 vs −2.28 mL/min/1.73 m^2/y, HR: 1.73 (1.10–2.37); P < .001) even though EMPEROR-Reduced enrolled patients with a lower eGFR at baseline.[5]

Of note, the EMPIRE-HF renal trial specifically assessed the short-term effect of empagliflozin on both congestion (using estimated plasma volume) and renal function in HFrEF. In this trial, empagliflozin was associated with a decline in measured GFR within 12 weeks of initiation along with a significant decline in estimated plasma volume and extracellular volume.[29] The early decline in measured GFR was expected due to hemodynamic effects, partly through the decongesting effect of SGLT2i. A similar initial decline in eGFR was noted within weeks of

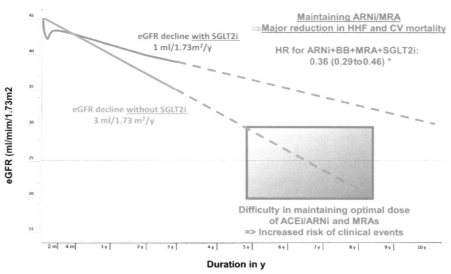

Fig. 1. Schemtic represntation of Renoprotective effects of SGLT2i on cardiovascular outcomes. ACEi, ACE inhibitors; ARNi, angiotensin receptor blocker/neprilysin inhibitor; BB, beta-blocker; CV, cardiovascular; HHF, hospitalization for heart failure; MRA, mineralocorticoid receptor antagonists. Dotted line represents extrapolated eGFR to longer follow-up than available evidence in DAPA-HF and EMPEROR-Reduced. (Tromp J, Ouwerkerk W, van Veldhuisen DJ, Hillege HL, Richards AM, van der Meer P, Anand IS, Lam CSP, Voors AA. A Systematic Review and Network Meta-Analysis of Pharmacological Treatment of Heart Failure with Reduced Ejection Fraction. JACC Heart Fail. 2022 Feb;10(2):73-84.)

SGLT2i initiation in DAPA-HF and EMPEROR-Reduced. This early drop was reversible after cessation of SGLT2i.[30] This drop was followed by a sustained improvement in eGFR slope in the SGLT2i group (compared with placebo) throughout the study period in both EMPEROR-Reduced and DAPA-HF, likely related to nonhemodynamic effects.

Trials assessing renal outcomes in patients with CKD and diabetes also conclusively show that SGLT2i are nephro-protective[6,31]: SGLT2i significantly reduced the risk of worsening renal function, end-stage kidney disease and renal death.[6,31] Furthermore, a post hoc analysis of DAPA-CKD in patients with baseline HF (n = 436) found that dapagliflozin reduced the composite of cardiorenal outcome by 42% (HR: 0.58 [0.37–0.91]).[32]

The above overall data underscore that SGLT2i reduce adverse renal outcomes and have substantial beneficial effects on preserving midterm renal function in HFrEF (**Fig. 1**).

Other clinically meaningful outcomes
Quality of Life: Short-term effects on quality of life were assessed in a moderately sized clinical trial (DEFINE-HF n = 263): a greater number of patients receiving dapagliflozin had a meaningful improvement (≥5 points) in the KCCQ-Overall Symptom Score (KCCQ-OSS) compared with patients receiving placebo (43% vs 33%) after 12 weeks of therapy.[33] Similarly, improvements in KCCQ-Total

Symptom Score were reported in the EMPULSE trial (mean difference 4.45 [0.32–8.59].[14] In the EMPERIAL-Reduced trial, there was no significant difference in KCCQ-TSS score between placebo and empagliflozin at the end of the 12 weeks. However, the median improvement in KCCQ-TSS was numerically higher by 3.13 (0.00–7.29) points in the empagliflozin group compared with placebo (change from baseline: 7.29 [–2.60 to 18.75] and 3.65 [–6.25 to 13.54], respectively) in patients with HFrEF,[34] which is within the same range of effect observed in the EMPULSE trial.

A midterm benefit in quality of life has been reported in both DAPA-HF and EMPEROR-Reduced trials, with SGLT2i being associated with better odds of meaningful improvement in KCCQ score (all components) (≥5-point-OSS odds ratio [OR]: 1.13[1.07–1.21] and 1.20 [1.05–1.37]) and lower odds of deterioration (≥5-point OSS OR 0.85 [0.80–0.91] and 0.75 [0.64–0.87], respectively).[35,36] In DAPA-HF, KCCQ-TSS score was 2.8 points higher in dapagliflozin versus placebo after 8 months of follow-up.[36] As point of reference, the improvement in KCCQ-OSS score was 1.1 after 8 months of treatment with sacubitril/valsartan.[37] Although no direct comparison on the improvement of quality of life between ARNi and SGLT2i has been performed, SGLT2i seem to provide a similar or greater overall improvement in quality of life.

Exercise tolerance: In 2 moderately sized, randomized double-blind trials, SUGAR-DM-HF and EMPIRE-HF, there was no significant difference in distance walked or physical activity between the SGLT2i and placebo group.[38,39] However, these neutral results could be due to relatively small sample size, relatively short-term outcome assessment, or the presence of comorbid conditions on which HF treatment has no effect. Exploratory studies have shown that SGLT2i may have a beneficial impact on exercise tolerance and cardiac oxygen consumption during exercise.[40,41] More evidence is needed to better understand the effect of SGLT2i on exercise tolerance.

Congestion: Adding SGLT2i to standard care significantly reduced congestion within a week in acutely decompensated HF.[42] SGLT2i reduced NT-pro-BNP levels in long-duration clinical trials (mean difference in pooled analysis: −194.0 [−249.9 to −138.0], I^2:61%).[43] In DEFINE-HF, dapagliflozin was not associated with a significant decline in NT-pro-BNP levels (1133 pg/dL [1036–1238] vs 1191 pg/dL [1089–1304], P = .43) at 12 weeks; however, more patients receiving SGLT2 had a meaningful reduction (≥20%) in NT-pro-BNP levels (OR: 1.9 [1.1–3.3]).[33] Even if decongestion effects exist, this did not translate into a significant decrease in loop diuretic dose in patients randomized to SGLT2i in DAPA-HF (mean furosemide-equivalent dose: 59.8 ± 109 vs 65.6 ± 104 mg at 12 months).[24] However, fewer patients receiving SGLT2i needed intensification of diuretic dose in both DAPA-HF (10.2% vs 14.2%, P < .001) and EMPEROR-Reduced trials (15.9% vs 22.2%) compared with placebo.[24,44]

Systolic function and ventricular remodeling: SGLT2i has been shown to improve some of the echocardiographic markers of left ventricular function.[38] In patients with HFrEF with diabetes/prediabetes, empagliflozin was associated with a decrease in left ventricular end-systolic (mean difference: −6.0 (−10.8 to −1.2) mL/m^2; P = .015) and end-diastolic volume index (mean difference: −8.2 (−13.7 to −2.6) mL/m^2; P = .004) in comparison to placebo after 36 weeks of treatment.[38] There was no significant change in LVEF (mean difference: 0.3 [−1.7–2.3]).[38]

Prevention of Heart Failure Onset in High-Risk Patients

SGLT2i seem to have pleiotropic effects on cardiovascular, metabolic, and renal systems.[45] A meta-analysis by Bhatia and colleagues estimated the relative and absolute effects of SGLT2i in preventing HF events in a broad spectrum of patients with cardiovascular or renal disease or diabetes.[46] Overall, SGLT2i reduced the risk of hospitalization for HF by 31% (HR 0.69 [0.64–0.74]). The absolute benefit from SGLT2i, however, was dependent on baseline risk: the number needed to treat to prevent one hospitalization for HF ranged from approximately 100 in CKD to 200 to 400 in high-risk diabetes. Given the high prevalence of diabetes and CKD, SGLT2i may have a large impact on the incidence of HF at the population level.

Diabetes: Trials performed in diabetes reported a significant and highly consistent reduction in hospitalization for HF with SGLT2i (EMPA-REG-Outcome HR: 0.65 (0.50–0.85), DECLARE-TIMI HR: 0.73 (0.61–0.88), CANVAS HR: 0.67 (0.52–0.87), and VERTIS-cardiovascular (VERTIS-CV) HR: 0.70 (0.54–0.90))[7–9,47] **(Table 2)**. A meta-analysis in patients with diabetes with or without atherosclerotic cardiovascular disease showed that hospitalization for HF was significantly reduced by SGLT2i but not by glucagon-like peptide-1 receptor agonists.[48]

A considerable amount of data on the efficacy of SGLT2i has emerged from large observational studies and population registries. The CVD-REAL and CVD-REAL2 multinational observational studies enrolled participants (n = 153,078/group and n = 235,064/group, respectively, after propensity score matching) who were newly initiated on SGLT2i and other glucose lowering drugs.[49,50] In CVD-REAL2, SGLT2i (vs other glucose lowering treatment) were associated with a significantly lower risk of hospitalization for HF (HR: 0.64 [0.50–0.82]). Similar findings were reported from CVD-REAL and the EASEL Population-Based Cohort Study.[50,51]

CKD: In patients with CKD, SGLT2i are associated with a reduced risk of cardiovascular outcomes. In a large, multicenter, randomized, double-blind trial (DAPA-CKD), dapagliflozin reduced the risk of cardiovascular death and hospitalization for HF by 29% (HR: 0.71 [0.55–0.92]) over a follow-up of 2.4 years.[6] Moreover, SGLT2i were seemingly equally effective in preventing hospitalizations for HF and urgent visits for HF in patients with both diabetes and CKD (HR = 0.67 [0.55–0.82]) in the SCORED trial in which only 20% of patients had a history of HF.[52]

Myocardial infarction: Patients with MI constitute a specific subgroup of interest in the setting of HF. Evidence regarding the efficacy of SGLT2i in patients with MI is relatively sparse. For the time being, SGLT2i have been evaluated in patients with acute MI in small–moderate-sized trials to assess whether they improve cardiac nerve activity.[53]

Table 2
Cardiovascular outcomes in patients receiving SGLT2i with Type 2 diabetes and CKD

Trial Name	Patient Population and Sub-population	Duration	N	HF at Baseline (n)	Objective	Endpoint	Results	Author, Year
EMPA-REG OUTCOME	Type 2 diabetes at high CV risk	3.1 y	7020	706	Examined the effects of empagliflozin, as compared with placebo, on CV morbidity and mortality in patients with type 2 diabetes at high risk for CV events receiving standard care	The primary composite outcome: death from CV causes, nonfatal MI, or nonfatal stroke HHF	HR: 0.86 (0.74–0.99) HR: 0.65 (0.50–0.85)	Zinman et al,[7] 2015
CANVAS	Type 2 diabetes and high CV risk	3.6 y	10,142	1461	Effects of treatment with canagliflozin on CV, renal, and safety outcomes	The primary composite outcome: death from CV causes, nonfatal MI, or nonfatal stroke HHF	HR: 0.86 (0.75–0.97). HR: 0.67(0.52–0.87)	Neal et al,[8] 2017
DECLARE-TIMI	Type 2 diabetes	4.2	17,160	1724	Evaluated the effects of dapagliflozin on CV and renal outcomes in patients who had or were at risk for atherosclerotic CV disease	The primary efficacy outcomes were MACE and a composite of CV death or HHF HHF	HR: 0.93 (0.84–1.03) HR: 0.73 (0.61–0.88)	Wiviott et al,[9] 2018
VERTIS-CV	Patients with type 2 diabetes and atherosclerotic CV disease	3.5 y	8246	1958	The long-term effects of ertugliflozin on CV and renal outcomes	The primary composite outcome: of death from CV causes, nonfatal MI, or nonfatal stroke HHF	HR: 0.97 (0.85–1.11) HR: 0.70 (0.54–0.90)	Cannon et al,[47] 2020

	Population	Duration	N	Objective	Outcome	Result	Reference
SCORED	Patients with diabetes with CKD with or without albuminuria	16 mo	10,584 3283	The efficacy and safety of sotagliflozin in preventing CV events in patients with diabetes with CKD with or without albuminuria	Composite of the total number of deaths from CV causes, HHF, and urgent visits for HF	HR:0.74 (0.63–0.88)	Bhatt et al,[52] 2021
					Total nb or hospitalizations for HF and urgent visits for HF	HR: 0.67 (0.55–0.82)	
CREDENCE	Type 2 diabetes and albuminuric CKD	2.62 y	4401	To assess the effects of canagliflozin on renal outcomes in patients with type 2 diabetes and albuminuric CKD	A composite of ESKD (dialysis, transplantation, or a sustained eGFR of <15 mL/min/1.73 m^2), a doubling of serum creatinine level, or death from renal or CV causes	The HR 0.70 (0.59–0.82)	Perkovic et al,[31] 2019
					HHF	HR 0.61 (0.47–0.80)	

Abbreviations: CKD, chronic kidney disease; CV, cardiovascular; ESKD, End-stage kidney disease; HF, heart failure; HHF, hospitalization for heart failure; HR, hazard ratio; MACE, major cardiovascular event; MI, myocardial infarction; nb, numer.

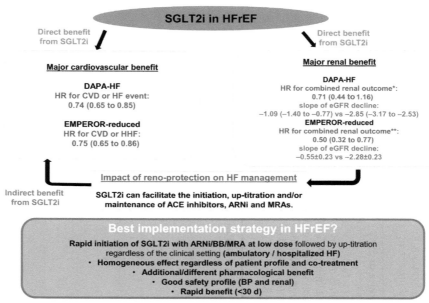

Fig. 2. Direct and indirect benefits of SGLT2i and possible implementation strategy in HFreF (* Refs.[4,28]; ** Ref.[5])

Safety Profile of Sodium-glucose cotransporter-2 inhibitors in Heart Failure with Reduced Ejection Fraction

SGLT2i seem to have an excellent safety profile in HFrEF. In most studies, the rate of adverse effects such as volume depletion, hypotension, and serious renal events with SGLT2i was similar to placebo in patients with HFrEF. However, the rate of genital tract infection may be higher with SGLT2i.[54] The risk of urinary tract infection seems to be higher in patients with diabetes in comparison to patients with HFrEF (ie, without diabetes).[4,7] In patients with acute HF with diabetes, sotagliflozin (which has a combined SGLT2i and SGLT1i effect) was associated with an increased risk of diarrhea and severe hypoglycemia.[13]

SGLT2i have relatively neutral effects on blood pressure and lack association with hypotension[55]: In patients with persistent low blood pressure, SGLT2i can consequently be continued.[55] In fact, when adjusted for placebo use, SGLT2i were associated with a slight early increase in systolic blood pressure in patients with blood pressure less than 110 mm Hg.[55]

Initiation of SGLT2i has been associated with an "eGFR dip" in the first few weeks of therapy, particularly in patients with advanced renal disease.[56,57] This initial dip in eGFR is expected and is similar to ACEi/ARBs.[58] This neither indicates AKI nor warrants discontinuation of therapy unless the dip is substantial (ie, >30% of eGFR and/or eGFR<25 mL/min). This initial change is reversible and, following this dip, SGLT2i have been found

significantly associated with reduced cardiovascular and renal outcomes.[30] Findings from large clinical trials actually suggest that SGLT2i have midterm renoprotective effects in HF, which ultimately is what matters most from a clinical perspective.

Additionally, a systematic review of observational studies identified that SGLT2i exposure was not associated with increased risk of AKI, urinary tract infection or fractures, albeit a possible risk of diabetic ketoacidosis in diabetes.[54]

Potential Impact of Renoprotective Properties of Sodium-glucose cotransporter-2 inhibitors in Heart Failure with Reduced Ejection Fraction

Nearly half of all patients with HFrEF have CKD. As CKD progresses, the volume overload/congestion becomes increasingly difficult to manage. The development of CKD is a known clinical variable associated with worse prognosis in HFrEF. In addition, worsening renal function and/or hyperkalemia is a major hurdle in maintaining HFrEF treatments.[58–60] Nevertheless, decreasing the dose of HFrEF drugs (eg, due to progressively declining renal function) is associated with poorer outcome.[61] ACEi and SGLT2i both have nephroprotective properties. However, with progressive renal failure, ACEi/ARNi are often withheld, which further exacerbates HF (**Fig. 2**). In contrast, SGLT2i can be prescribed to patients with eGFR as low as 20 mL/min/1.73 m.[2] More importantly, SGLT2i slow the progression of CKD in HFrEF, thereby facilitating the maintenance of optimal doses of HF drugs.[3] The continued prescription of these drugs at optimal dose is highly likely to translate into long-term clinical benefits. As mentioned above, among patients receiving MRA at baseline, SGLT2i were associated with a lower frequency of MRA discontinuation compared with placebo in the EMPEROR-Reduced trial.[25] In turn, maintaining MRA will also further enhance the impact of SGLT2i because it has been estimated that a comprehensive treatment with all 4 drugs (ARNi + ß-blocker + MRA + SGLT2i) reduces cardiovascular death or hospitalization for HF by 62% in comparison with limited conventional therapy (ACEi/ARBs + ß-blocker),[62] the latter being more likely to be used in patients with impaired renal function. Yet, this long-term benefit cannot be derived from trials (since having a relatively short follow-up).

Fig. 1 schematically illustrates the impact of SGLT2i renoprotective effects on drug prescription and subsequent prognosis in HFrEF.

Implementation of Sodium-glucose cotransporter-2 inhibitors in Heart Failure with Reduced Ejection Fraction

The present guidelines recommend SGLT2i in all patients with HFrEF combined with the foundational therapy consisting of ACEi/ARNi, ß-blocker, and MRAs.[1,2] However, the guidelines do not suggest any specific sequence of drug initiation and/or up-titration. In the ESC 2016 guidelines for HF, a sequential approach for HF drug optimization was recommended,[63] which could lead to a substantial delay in the initiation of life-saving therapies. Several HF experts propose a more fast-track approach that allows early initiation of SGLT2i to reduce the subsequent risk of CV death and/or hospitalization and for better tolerability of MRAs and ACEi.[64,65] From a pharmacologic standpoint, different classes of HFrEF treatments are more likely to have additive benefits as opposed to maximizing one particular drug class. In addition, evidence of benefits seemed very early and were significant within 30 days in the DAPA-HF trial (HR: 0.51[0.28–0.94] at 28 days of treatment).[4,66] McMurray et al. and Greene and colleagues accordingly suggest that it may be more beneficial to initiate all drugs at low dose concomitantly (or within a short time-frame) rather than a "sequential" sequence (up-titrating one and then adding the next drug).[64,65] In addition, given the excellent safety profile of SGLT2i, their initiation may actually be better tolerated than up-titration of another class (eg, in a patient with borderline BP and heart rate, it would be actually easier to add SGLT2i than increase beta-blockers).

Knowledge Gaps

SGLT2i may have a class effect with no substantial difference in efficacy across drugs. However, a recent network meta-analysis indicates that empagliflozin, canagliflozin, and dapagliflozin are equally effective in improving worsening HF, whereas empagliflozin was superior to other SGLT2i in reducing all-cause and cardiovascular death.[67] However, these results may emerge from differences in the trials per se rather than differences in actual SGLT2i effects. More direct comparison studies will be needed to determine whether a specific SGLT2 inhibitor should be used in a given patient to maximize its benefit.

Several mechanisms mediating SGLT2i activity have been suggested such as osmotic diuresis and natriuresis leading to decongestion, improved cardiac metabolism, improved myocardial efficiency, reduced sympathetic overdrive, and reduced oxidative stress and inflammation.[68] However, key mechanisms underlying SGLT2i efficacy have yet to be clearly elucidated.

SGLT2i are effective in reducing adverse outcomes regardless of background therapy. However, the best implementation strategy for prescribing SGLT2i in HFrEF needs to be outlined. A fundamental question that remains is "should SGLT2 inhibitors be initiated at very early stages of HFrEF?". Dedicated trials should test whether a fast-track implementation strategy of SGLT2i provides additional benefits to a conventional approach of initiating and up-titrating the foundational therapy of ACEi/ARBs, ß-blocker, and MRAs and subsequently adding SGLT2i.[64,65] Current guidelines leave the decision, to physicians on how SGLT2 inhibitor should be initiated in de novo HF, especially in the setting of acute HF.

Additional data is, moreover, needed on whether SGLT2i are equally effective in preventing HF onset in post-MI patients. The ongoing DAPA-MI (NCT04564742) and EMPACT-MI (NCT04509674) trials should clarify the effect of SGLT2i in patients with acute MI.

SUMMARY

SGLT2i have a homogeneous/pleiotropic benefit in cardiovascular medicine, including HFrEF. The cardio-renal protective effect of SGLT2i is a major evolution in the treatment of HFrEF. How to best implement this important therapeutic breakthrough is to be better determined. However, given the very rapid impact of SGLT2i on outcome and their good safety profile, an early introduction of these drugs in most patients with HFrEF seems to be advisable.

CLINICS CARE POINTS

- Sodium-glucose cotransporter-2 inhibitors (SGLT2i) are safe and effective in heart failure with reduced ejection fraction with or without diabetes and/or with or without chronic kidney disease (CKD).
- Given the rapid efficacy of SGLT2i, physicians should target an early initiation of these drugs to reduce the risk of adverse cardiovascular and renal outcome.
- At SGLT2i initiation, patients must be informed on the risk of urinary tract/genital infection and advised on perineal hygiene.
- At SGLT2i initiation in patients with diabetes, dose reduction of insulin and sulfonylureas should be considered to avoid the risk of hypoglycemia.
- Before initiating SGLT2i in patients with impaired renal function/CKD, renal function and volume status must be assessed. If hypovolemia is present, then it must be corrected before initiating SGLT2i.
- Renal function monitoring after SLGT2i initiation may be required in patients with CKD because of initial eGFR dip. Dose adjustments/temporary cessation of SGLT2i may be considered if eGFR dip is substantial ($\geq$30% decline of eGFR).

DISCLOSURE

Dr N. Girerd reports personal fees from AstraZeneca, personal fees from Bayer, personal fees from Boehringer, personal fees from Lilly, personal fees from Novartis, personal fees from Vifor, outside the submitted work.

REFERENCES

1. McDonagh TA, Metra M, Adamo M, et al. ESC Guidelines for the diagnosis and treatment of acute and chronic heart failure: Developed by the Task Force for the diagnosis and treatment of acute and chronic heart failure of the European Society of Cardiology (ESC) With the special contribution of the Heart Failure Association (HFA) of the ESC. Eur Heart J 2021;42(36):3599–726. https://doi.org/10.1093/eurheartj/ehab368.
2. Maddox TM, Januzzi JL, Allen LA, et al. 2021 Update to the 2017 ACC Expert Consensus Decision Pathway for Optimization of Heart Failure Treatment: Answers to 10 Pivotal Issues About Heart Failure With Reduced Ejection Fraction. J Am Coll Cardiol 2021;77(6):772–810. https://doi.org/10.1016/j.jacc.2020.11.022.
3. Rossignol P. A Step Forward Toward a New Treatment Paradigm in the Cardiorenal Continuum. JACC: Heart Failure 2021;9(11):821–3.
4. McMurray JJV, Solomon SD, Inzucchi SE, et al. Dapagliflozin in Patients with Heart Failure and Reduced Ejection Fraction. N Engl J Med 2019;381(21):1995–2008. https://doi.org/10.1056/NEJMoa1911303.
5. Packer M, Anker SD, Butler J, et al. Cardiovascular and Renal Outcomes with Empagliflozin in Heart Failure. N Engl J Med 2020;383(15):1413–24. https://doi.org/10.1056/NEJMoa2022190.
6. Heerspink HJL, Stefánsson BV, Correa-Rotter R, et al. Dapagliflozin in Patients with Chronic Kidney Disease. N Engl J Med 2020;383(15):1436–46. https://doi.org/10.1056/NEJMoa2024816.
7. Zinman B, Wanner C, Lachin JM, et al. Empagliflozin, Cardiovascular Outcomes, and Mortality in Type 2 Diabetes. N Engl J Med 2015;373(22):2117–28. https://doi.org/10.1056/NEJMoa1504720.
8. Neal B, Perkovic V, Mahaffey KW, et al. Canagliflozin and Cardiovascular and Renal Events in Type 2 Diabetes. New Engl J Med 2017;377(7):644–57. https://doi.org/10.1056/NEJMoa1611925.
9. Wiviott SD, Raz I, Bonaca MP, et al. Dapagliflozin and Cardiovascular Outcomes in Type 2 Diabetes. N Engl J Med 2019;380(4):347–57. https://doi.org/10.1056/NEJMoa1812389.
10. McMurray JJV. EMPEROR-Reduced: confirming sodium-glucose co-transporter 2 inhibitors as an essential treatment for patients with heart failure with reduced ejection fraction. Eur J Heart Fail 2020;22(11):1987–90. https://doi.org/10.1002/ejhf.2006.
11. Zannad F, Ferreira JP, Pocock SJ, et al. SGLT2 inhibitors in patients with heart failure with reduced ejection fraction: a meta-analysis of the EMPEROR-Reduced and DAPA-HF trials. Lancet 2020;396(10254):819–29. https://doi.org/10.1016/s0140-6736(20)31824-9.
12. Damman K, Beusekamp JC, Boorsma EM, et al. Randomized, double-blind, placebo-controlled, multicentre pilot study on the effects of empagliflozin on clinical outcomes in patients with acute decompensated heart failure (EMPA-RESPONSE-AHF). Eur J Heart Fail 2020;22(4):713–22. https://doi.org/10.1002/ejhf.1713.
13. Bhatt DL, Szarek M, Steg PG, et al. Sotagliflozin in Patients with Diabetes and Recent Worsening Heart Failure. N Engl J Med 2021;384(2):117–28. https://doi.org/10.1056/NEJMoa2030183.
14. Voors AA, Angermann CE, Teerlink JR, et al. The SGLT2 inhibitor empagliflozin in patients hospitalized for acute heart failure: a multinational randomized trial. Nat Med 2022;28:568–74. https://doi.org/10.1038/s41591-021-01659-1.

15. Butt JH, Nicolau JC, Verma S, et al. Efficacy and safety of dapagliflozin according to aetiology in heart failure with reduced ejection fraction: insights from the DAPA-HF trial. Eur J Heart Fail 2021; 23(4):601–13. https://doi.org/10.1002/ejhf.2124.

16. Anker SD, Butler J, Filippatos G, et al. Effect of Empagliflozin on Cardiovascular and Renal Outcomes in Patients With Heart Failure by Baseline Diabetes Status: Results From the EMPEROR-Reduced Trial. Circulation 2021;143(4):337–49. https://doi.org/10.1161/circulationaha.120.051824.

17. Zelniker TA, Raz I, Mosenzon O, et al. Effect of Dapagliflozin on Cardiovascular Outcomes According to Baseline Kidney Function and Albuminuria Status in Patients With Type 2 Diabetes: A Prespecified Secondary Analysis of a Randomized Clinical Trial. JAMA Cardiol 2021;6(7):801–10. https://doi.org/10.1001/jamacardio.2021.0660.

18. Zannad F, Ferreira JP, Pocock SJ, et al. Cardiac and Kidney Benefits of Empagliflozin in Heart Failure Across the Spectrum of Kidney Function: Insights From EMPEROR-Reduced. Circulation 2021;143(4):310–21. https://doi.org/10.1161/circulationaha.120.051685.

19. Dewan P, Docherty KF, Bengtsson O, et al. Effects of dapagliflozin in heart failure with reduced ejection fraction and chronic obstructive pulmonary disease: an analysis of DAPA-HF. Eur J Heart Fail 2021;23(4):632–43. https://doi.org/10.1002/ejhf.2083.

20. Martinez FA, Serenelli M, Nicolau JC, et al. Efficacy and Safety of Dapagliflozin in Heart Failure With Reduced Ejection Fraction According to Age: Insights From DAPA-HF. Circulation 2020;141(2):100–11. https://doi.org/10.1161/circulationaha.119.044133.

21. Yeoh SE, Dewan P, Jhund PS, et al. Patient Characteristics, Clinical Outcomes, and Effect of Dapagliflozin in Relation to Duration of Heart Failure: Is It Ever Too Late to Start a New Therapy? Circ Heart Fail 2020;13(12):e007879. https://doi.org/10.1161/circheartfailure.120.007879.

22. Petrie MC, Verma S, Docherty KF, et al. Effect of Dapagliflozin on Worsening Heart Failure and Cardiovascular Death in Patients With Heart Failure With and Without Diabetes. JAMA 2020;323(14):1353–68. https://doi.org/10.1001/jama.2020.1906.

23. Packer M, Anker SD, Butler J, et al. Influence of neprilysin inhibition on the efficacy and safety of empagliflozin in patients with chronic heart failure and a reduced ejection fraction: the EMPEROR-Reduced trial. Eur Heart J 2021;42(6):671–80. https://doi.org/10.1093/eurheartj/ehaa968.

24. Jackson AM, Dewan P, Anand IS, et al. Dapagliflozin and Diuretic Use in Patients With Heart Failure and Reduced Ejection Fraction in DAPA-HF. Circulation 2020;142(11):1040–54. https://doi.org/10.1161/circulationaha.120.047077.

25. Ferreira JP, Zannad F, Pocock SJ, et al. Interplay of Mineralocorticoid Receptor Antagonists and Empagliflozin in Heart Failure: EMPEROR-Reduced. J Am Coll Cardiol 2021;77(11):1397–407. https://doi.org/10.1016/j.jacc.2021.01.044.

26. Solomon SD, Jhund PS, Claggett BL, et al. Effect of Dapagliflozin in Patients With HFrEF Treated With Sacubitril/Valsartan: The DAPA-HF Trial. JACC Heart Fail 2020;8(10):811–8. https://doi.org/10.1016/j.jchf.2020.04.008.

27. Hsiao FC, Lin CP, Tung YC, et al. Combining sodium-glucose cotransporter 2 inhibitors and angiotensin receptor-neprilysin inhibitors in heart failure patients with reduced ejection fraction and diabetes mellitus: A multi-institutional study. Int J Cardiol 2021;330:91–7. https://doi.org/10.1016/j.ijcard.2021.02.035.

28. Jhund PS, Solomon SD, Docherty KF, et al. Efficacy of Dapagliflozin on Renal Function and Outcomes in Patients With Heart Failure With Reduced Ejection Fraction: Results of DAPA-HF. Circulation 2021; 143(4):298–309. https://doi.org/10.1161/circulationaha.120.050391.

29. Jensen J, Omar M, Kistorp C, et al. Effects of empagliflozin on estimated extracellular volume, estimated plasma volume, and measured glomerular filtration rate in patients with heart failure (Empire HF Renal): a prespecified substudy of a double-blind, randomised, placebo-controlled trial. Lancet Diabetes Endocrinol 2021;9(2):106–16. https://doi.org/10.1016/s2213-8587(20)30382-x.

30. Wanner C, Inzucchi SE, Lachin JM, et al. Empagliflozin and Progression of Kidney Disease in Type 2 Diabetes. N Engl J Med 2016;375(4):323–34. https://doi.org/10.1056/NEJMoa1515920.

31. Perkovic V, Jardine MJ, Neal B, et al. Canagliflozin and Renal Outcomes in Type 2 Diabetes and Nephropathy. N Engl J Med 2019;380(24):2295–306. https://doi.org/10.1056/NEJMoa1811744.

32. McMurray JJV, Wheeler DC, Stefánsson BV, et al. Effects of Dapagliflozin in Patients With Kidney Disease, With and Without Heart Failure. JACC Heart Fail 2021. https://doi.org/10.1016/j.jchf.2021.06.017.

33. Nassif ME, Windsor SL, Tang F, et al. Dapagliflozin Effects on Biomarkers, Symptoms, and Functional Status in Patients With Heart Failure With Reduced Ejection Fraction: The DEFINE-HF Trial. Circulation 2019;140(18):1463–76. https://doi.org/10.1161/circulationaha.119.042929.

34. Abraham WT, Lindenfeld J, Ponikowski P, et al. Effect of empagliflozin on exercise ability and symptoms in heart failure patients with reduced and preserved ejection fraction, with and without type 2 diabetes. Eur Heart J 2021;42(6):700–10. https://doi.org/10.1093/eurheartj/ehaa943.

35. Butler J, Anker SD, Filippatos G, et al. Empagliflozin and health-related quality of life outcomes in patients with heart failure with reduced ejection

fraction: the EMPEROR-Reduced trial. Eur Heart J 2021;42(13):1203–12. https://doi.org/10.1093/eurheartj/ehaa1007.

36. Kosiborod MN, Jhund PS, Docherty KF, et al. Effects of Dapagliflozin on Symptoms, Function, and Quality of Life in Patients With Heart Failure and Reduced Ejection Fraction: Results From the DAPA-HF Trial. Circulation 2020;141(2):90–9. https://doi.org/10.1161/circulationaha.119.044138.

37. Lewis EF, Claggett BL, McMurray JJV, et al. Health-Related Quality of Life Outcomes in PARADIGM-HF. Circ Heart Fail 2017;10(8). https://doi.org/10.1161/circheartfailure.116.003430.

38. Lee MMY, Brooksbank KJM, Wetherall K, et al. Effect of Empagliflozin on Left Ventricular Volumes in Patients With Type 2 Diabetes, or Prediabetes, and Heart Failure With Reduced Ejection Fraction (SUGAR-DM-HF). Circulation 2021;143(6):516–25. https://doi.org/10.1161/circulationaha.120.052186.

39. Jensen J, Omar M, Kistorp C, et al. Twelve weeks of treatment with empagliflozin in patients with heart failure and reduced ejection fraction: A double-blinded, randomized, and placebo-controlled trial. Am Heart J 2020;228:47–56. https://doi.org/10.1016/j.ahj.2020.07.011.

40. Núñez J, Palau P, Domínguez E, et al. Early effects of empagliflozin on exercise tolerance in patients with heart failure: A pilot study. Clin Cardiol 2018;41(4):476–80. https://doi.org/10.1002/clc.22899.

41. Carbone S, Canada JM, Billingsley HE, et al. Effects of empagliflozin on cardiorespiratory fitness and significant interaction of loop diuretics. Diabetes Obes Metab 2018;20(8):2014–8. https://doi.org/10.1111/dom.13309.

42. Tamaki S, Yamada T, Watanabe T, et al. Effect of Empagliflozin as an Add-On Therapy on Decongestion and Renal Function in Patients With Diabetes Hospitalized for Acute Decompensated Heart Failure: A Prospective Randomized Controlled Study. Circ Heart Fail 2021;14(3):e007048. https://doi.org/10.1161/circheartfailure.120.007048.

43. Chambergo-Michilot D, Tauma-Arrué A, Loli-Guevara S. Effects and safety of SGLT2 inhibitors compared to placebo in patients with heart failure: A systematic review and meta-analysis. Int J Cardiol Heart Vasc 2021;32:100690. https://doi.org/10.1016/j.ijcha.2020.100690.

44. Packer M, Anker SD, Butler J, et al. Effect of Empagliflozin on the Clinical Stability of Patients With Heart Failure and a Reduced Ejection Fraction: The EMPEROR-Reduced Trial. Circulation 2021;143(4):326–36. https://doi.org/10.1161/circulationaha.120.051783.

45. Patel DK, Strong J. The Pleiotropic Effects of Sodium-Glucose Cotransporter-2 Inhibitors: Beyond the Glycemic Benefit. Diabetes Ther 2019;10(5):1771–92. https://doi.org/10.1007/s13300-019-00686-z.

46. Bhatia K, Jain V, Gupta K, et al. Prevention of heart failure events with sodium-glucose co-transporter 2 inhibitors across a spectrum of cardio-renal-metabolic risk. Eur J Heart Fail 2021;23(6):1002–8. https://doi.org/10.1002/ejhf.2135.

47. Cannon CP, Pratley R, Dagogo-Jack S, et al. Cardiovascular Outcomes with Ertugliflozin in Type 2 Diabetes. N Engl J Med 2020;383(15):1425–35. https://doi.org/10.1056/NEJMoa2004967.

48. Zelniker TA, Wiviott SD, Raz I, et al. Comparison of the Effects of Glucagon-Like Peptide Receptor Agonists and Sodium-Glucose Cotransporter 2 Inhibitors for Prevention of Major Adverse Cardiovascular and Renal Outcomes in Type 2 Diabetes Mellitus. Circulation 2019;139(17):2022–31. https://doi.org/10.1161/circulationaha.118.038868.

49. Kosiborod M, Lam CSP, Kohsaka S, et al. Cardiovascular Events Associated With SGLT-2 Inhibitors Versus Other Glucose-Lowering Drugs: The CVD-REAL 2 Study. J Am Coll Cardiol 2018;71(23):2628–39. https://doi.org/10.1016/j.jacc.2018.03.009.

50. Cavender MA, Norhammar A, Birkeland KI, et al. SGLT-2 Inhibitors and Cardiovascular Risk: An Analysis of CVD-REAL. J Am Coll Cardiol 2018;71(22):2497–506. https://doi.org/10.1016/j.jacc.2018.01.085.

51. Udell JA, Yuan Z, Rush T, et al. Cardiovascular Outcomes and Risks After Initiation of a Sodium Glucose Cotransporter 2 Inhibitor: Results From the EASEL Population-Based Cohort Study (Evidence for Cardiovascular Outcomes With Sodium Glucose Cotransporter 2 Inhibitors in the Real World). Circulation 2018;137(14):1450–9. https://doi.org/10.1161/circulationaha.117.031227.

52. Bhatt DL, Szarek M, Pitt B, et al. Sotagliflozin in Patients with Diabetes and Chronic Kidney Disease. N Engl J Med 2021;384(2):129–39. https://doi.org/10.1056/NEJMoa2030186.

53. Shimizu W, Kubota Y, Hoshika Y, et al. Effects of empagliflozin versus placebo on cardiac sympathetic activity in acute myocardial infarction patients with type 2 diabetes mellitus: the EMBODY trial. Cardiovasc Diabetol 2020;19(1):148. https://doi.org/10.1186/s12933-020-01127-z.

54. Caparrotta TM, Greenhalgh AM, Osinski K, et al. Sodium-Glucose Co-Transporter 2 Inhibitors (SGLT2i) Exposure and Outcomes in Type 2 Diabetes: A Systematic Review of Population-Based Observational Studies. Diabetes Ther 2021;12(4):991–1028. https://doi.org/10.1007/s13300-021-01004-2.

55. Böhm M, Anker SD, Butler J, et al. Empagliflozin Improves Cardiovascular and Renal Outcomes in Heart Failure Irrespective of Systolic Blood Pressure.

J Am Coll Cardiol 2021;78(13):1337–48. https://doi.org/10.1016/j.jacc.2021.07.049.

56. Wanner C, Heerspink HJL, Zinman B, et al. Empagliflozin and Kidney Function Decline in Patients with Type 2 Diabetes: A Slope Analysis from the EMPA-REG OUTCOME Trial. J Am Soc Nephrol 2018;29(11):2755–69. https://doi.org/10.1681/asn.2018010103.

57. Oshima M, Jardine MJ, Agarwal R, et al. Insights from CREDENCE trial indicate an acute drop in estimated glomerular filtration rate during treatment with canagliflozin with implications for clinical practice. Kidney Int 2021;99(4):999–1009. https://doi.org/10.1016/j.kint.2020.10.042.

58. Mewton N, Girerd N, Boffa JJ, et al. Practical management of worsening renal function in outpatients with heart failure and reduced ejection fraction: Statement from a panel of multidisciplinary experts and the Heart Failure Working Group of the French Society of Cardiology. Arch Cardiovasc Dis 2020;113(10):660–70. https://doi.org/10.1016/j.acvd.2020.03.018.

59. Shirazian S, Grant CD, Mujeeb S, et al. Underprescription of renin-angiotensin system blockers in moderate to severe chronic kidney disease. Am J Med Sci 2015;349(6):510–5. https://doi.org/10.1097/maj.0000000000000475.

60. Trevisan M, de Deco P, Xu H, et al. Incidence, predictors and clinical management of hyperkalaemia in new users of mineralocorticoid receptor antagonists. Eur J Heart Fail 2018;20(8):1217–26. https://doi.org/10.1002/ejhf.1199.

61. Ouwerkerk W, Voors AA, Anker SD, et al. Determinants and clinical outcome of uptitration of ACE-inhibitors and beta-blockers in patients with heart failure: a prospective European study. Eur Heart J 2017;38(24):1883–90. https://doi.org/10.1093/eurheartj/ehx026.

62. Vaduganathan M, Claggett BL, Jhund PS, et al. Estimating lifetime benefits of comprehensive disease-modifying pharmacological therapies in patients with heart failure with reduced ejection fraction: a comparative analysis of three randomised controlled trials. Lancet 2020;396(10244):121–8. https://doi.org/10.1016/s0140-6736(20)30748-0.

63. Ponikowski P, Voors AA, Anker SD, et al. ESC Guidelines for the diagnosis and treatment of acute and chronic heart failure: The Task Force for the diagnosis and treatment of acute and chronic heart failure of the European Society of Cardiology (ESC) Developed with the special contribution of the Heart Failure Association (HFA) of the ESC. Eur Heart J 2016;37(27):2129–200. https://doi.org/10.1093/eurheartj/ehw128.

64. McMurray JJV, Packer M. How Should We Sequence the Treatments for Heart Failure and a Reduced Ejection Fraction?: A Redefinition of Evidence-Based Medicine. Circ 2021;143(9):875–7. https://doi.org/10.1161/CIRCULATIONAHA.120.052926.

65. Greene SJ, Butler J, Fonarow GC. Simultaneous or Rapid Sequence Initiation of Quadruple Medical Therapy for Heart Failure-Optimizing Therapy With the Need for Speed. JAMA Cardiol 2021;6(7):743–4. https://doi.org/10.1001/jamacardio.2021.0496.

66. Berg DD, Jhund PS, Docherty KF, et al. Time to Clinical Benefit of Dapagliflozin and Significance of Prior Heart Failure Hospitalization in Patients With Heart Failure With Reduced Ejection Fraction. JAMA Cardiol 2021;6(5):499–507. https://doi.org/10.1001/jamacardio.2020.7585.

67. Täger T, Atar D, Agewall S, et al. Comparative efficacy of sodium-glucose cotransporter-2 inhibitors (SGLT2i) for cardiovascular outcomes in type 2 diabetes: a systematic review and network meta-analysis of randomised controlled trials. Heart Fail Rev 2021;26(6):1421–35. https://doi.org/10.1007/s10741-020-09954-8.

68. Zelniker TA, Braunwald E. Mechanisms of Cardiorenal Effects of Sodium-Glucose Cotransporter 2 Inhibitors: JACC State-of-the-Art Review. J Am Coll Cardiol 2020;75(4):422–34. https://doi.org/10.1016/j.jacc.2019.11.031.

SGLT2 Inhibitors and Heart Failure with Preserved Ejection Fraction

Pardeep S. Jhund, BSc, MBChB, MSc, PhD

KEYWORDS

- Heart failure with preserved ejection fraction • Heart failure with reduced ejection fraction
- Chronic kidney disease • Diabetes • SGLT2 inhibitors • Hospitalizations • Mortality

KEY POINTS

- Secondary analyses of the trials of SGLT2 inhibitors in patients with type 2 diabetes suggested a benefit of this class of drugs in heart failure with preserved ejection fraction (HFPEF).
- The EMPEROR-Preserved trial randomized patients with HFPEF to empagliflozin or placebo.
- Empagliflozin reduced the risk of cardiovascular (CV) death or hospitalization for heart failure by 21%, mainly due to a reduction in hospitalization for heart failure with no effect on CV mortality.
- Empagliflozin is the first drug to reduce the primary outcome in a trial of patients with HFPEF and more trials with other SGLT2 inhibitors in patients with HFPEF are due to conclude.
- SGLT2 inhibitors will become the new standard of care in HFPEF.

Since the publication of the EMPA-REG-Outcome trial, there has been huge interest in the potential benefit of sodium-glucose co-transporter 2 (SGLT2) inhibitors in patients with heart failure.[1] The dramatic results of EMPA-REG-Outcome trial demonstrated a reduction in heart failure hospitalizations with the SGLT2 inhibitor empagliflozin, and whether these drugs would be of benefit in patients with heart failure became a subject of much investigation. Several other trials of SGLT2 inhibitors in patients with type 2 diabetes soon followed,[2–5] replicating the results of the EMPA-REG-Outcome trial. More recently, there have been 2 large placebo-controlled randomized trials of SGLT2 inhibitors (dapagliflozin and then empagliflozin), which have reported a reduction in morbidity and mortality in patients with heart failure with reduced ejection fraction (HFREF).[6,7] However, a large proportion of the population with heart failure have heart failure with preserved ejection fraction (HFPEF) and what was previously known as midrange ejection fraction heart failure or what is now recognized as mildly reduced ejection fraction heart failure. In some epidemiologic studies, up to 50% of patients presenting with heart failure have an ejection fraction of more than 40%.[8] This leaves a large proportion of patients who have currently not been eligible for the treatment with SGLT2 inhibitor based on current guidelines.[9] This review will examine the efficacy of SGLT2 inhibitors in patients with HFPEF.

DIABETES, HEART FAILURE WITH PRESERVED EJECTION FRACTION, AND SGLT2 INHIBITORS

There have been several trials of SGLT2 inhibitors in patients with type 2 diabetes.[1–5] When these trials were initiated, the benefit of SGLT2 inhibitors on heart failure hospitalizations, and the degree to which these drugs would reduce the risk of heart failure hospitalizations, was not anticipated. As such, when patients were enrolled into these trials, detailed information about left ejection fraction (LVEF) was not always collected. However, several investigators did record LVEF and all recorded whether a patient had a history of heart

British Heart Foundation Cardiovascular Research Centre, Institute of Cardiovascular and Medical Sciences, University of Glasgow, 126 University Place, Glasgow G12 8TA, United Kingdom
E-mail address: pardeep.jhund@glasgow.ac.uk

Heart Failure Clin 18 (2022) 579–586
https://doi.org/10.1016/j.hfc.2022.03.010
1551-7136/22/© 2022 Elsevier Inc. All rights reserved.

failure and therefore were able to provide some insights into the potential benefit of SGLT2 inhibitors in patients with HFPEF. The EMPA-REG Outcome trial was the first to report the benefit of SGLT2 inhibitors in type 2 diabetes. Data on LVEF was not collected, but the efficacy of empagliflozin was similar in those with and without heart failure.[10] The CANVAS program, with the SGLT2 inhibitor canagliflozin, in patients with type 2 diabetes and at high risk for developing cardiovascular (CV) disease included 10,142 patients and did not collect LVEF data. The investigators did report that the benefit of canagliflozin was greater in those with a history of heart failure.[3] In a trial of canagliflozin (this time enrolling those with kidney disease caused by type 2 diabetes), a reduction in kidney and CV events in those with a prior history of heart failure at baseline (15%) was observed in those randomized to canagliflozin.[4] However, it was not until an analysis of the DECLARE-TIMI 58 trial with the SGLT2 inhibitor dapagliflozin that some insight into the potential benefit of SGLT2 inhibitors in HFPEF in particular was reported[11] (**Fig. 1**). In the trial, there were 17,160 patients enrolled, and of those, 1987 (12%) had a history of heart failure. Of this group, 671 (3.9%) had an ejection fraction of less than 45% and 1316 (7.7%) had heart failure without reduced ejection fraction including 808 with ejection fraction of 45% or greater. Although the treatment benefit with dapagliflozin seemed to be greater in those with HFREF (hazard ratio [HR] 0.62 95%CI 0.45–0.86) than those with HFPEF (HR 0.88 95%CI 0.66–1.17), there was no interaction between the treatment and type of heart failure (P for interaction = 0.45). In keeping with a subsequent analysis of the DAPA-HF trial,[12] the benefit of dapagliflozin in those with HFREF was observed very early during follow-up (almost immediately), whereas in those with HFPEF, the divergence in the rates of CV death or heart failure (HF) hospitalization occurred around 1 year of follow-up. After these seminal trials of SGLT2 inhibitors in patients with type 2 diabetes, the VERTIS-CV trial reported.[5] This was a placebo-controlled trial of ertugliflozin in patients with type 2 diabetes and established atherosclerotic CV disease. In this trial, the benefit of ertugliflozin was similar in those with and without heart failure and in those with an ejection fraction of more than 45% versus those with an ejection fraction 45% or greater. Before the results of a trial of SGLT2 inhibitors in patients with HFPEF, 2 other trials in patients with type 2 diabetes provided further insight into whether these drugs may be beneficial in HFPEF. A trial of an SGLT1/2 inhibitor, sotagliflozin, the SOLOIST-WHF trial,[13] randomized patients with type 2 diabetes and decompensated heart failure to sotagliflozin or placebo. Randomization was stratified according to LVEF allowing subsequent examination of the HFPEF group. Unfortunately, this trial was terminated early due to loss of funding, but overall, there was a benefit of sotagliflozin on the primary composite endpoint of CV death and total heart failure hospitalizations. However, despite the early termination of the trial, there were substantial number of events after 1222 patients were enrolled, of which 21% had HFPEF. The authors reported that there was no difference in the benefit of sotagliflozin according to HF type. At the same time, the SCORED trial[14] was published, again using sotagliflozin; but in this trial in patients with type 2 diabetes, high CV risk, and chronic kidney disease, several patients had heart failure. The benefit again was the same in those with HFREF and HFPEF. In a presentation of a combined analysis of SOLOIST and SCORED, the benefit of sotagliflozin was clear in the combined HFPEF subgroups from both trials with no evidence of interaction by ejection fraction (P for interaction = 0.33[15]; see **Fig. 1**). However, given that both trials were terminated early and that these were not primary analyses, these data had to be viewed with caution until adequately powered trials in patients with HFPEF could be completed.

EMPAGLIFLOZIN AND HEART FAILURE WITH PRESERVED EJECTION FRACTION

Having observed that SGLT2 inhibitors improved outcomes in the HFREF population with and without type 2 diabetes in 2 large randomized trials,[6,7] combined with the exploratory analyses of trials in patients with type 2 diabetes, the results of an adequately powered trial in HFPEF with and SGLT2 inhibitor were keenly awaited. Trials of pharmacotherapies in HFPEF had been neutral and the most recent drug to demonstrate a benefit in HFREF, sacubitril/valsartan, was tested in a population with HFPEF, and again, the result of the primary outcome was neutral.[16] The EMPEROR-Preserved trial was a multicenter, randomized, double-blind, placebo-controlled trial designed to evaluate whether empagliflozin would improve morbidity and mortality in patients with HFPEF.[17,18] The trial enrolled patients who have had heart failure for at least 3 months (in New York Heart Association Class II, III, or IV) and in whom LVEF was greater than 40% at its most recent assessment with no prior measurement of ejection fraction being 40% or lower. They were required to have elevated N-terminal pro-brain natriuretic peptide (NT-proBNP) levels (ie, >300 pg/mL in patients without atrial fibrillation and >900 pg/mL in patients

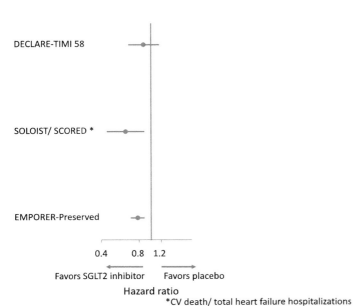

DECLARE-TIMI 58

SOLOIST/ SCORED *

EMPORER-Preserved

0.4   0.8 1.2

Favors SGLT2 inhibitor   Favors placebo

Hazard ratio

*CV death/ total heart failure hospitalizations

Fig. 1. Effect of SGLT2 inhibitors on CV death or heart failure (HF) hospitalization in trials of SGLT2 inhibitors in patients with type 2 diabetes where information on HFPEF was available versus the treatment estimate of empagliflozin reported from EMPEROR-Preserved. [a]CV death/total heart failure hospitalizations.

with atrial fibrillation) and to show evidence of structural changes in the heart (as evidenced by increases in left atrial size or left ventricular mass) on echocardiography or a documented hospitalization for heart failure within 12 months of screening.

The primary end point of EMPEROR-Preserved was a composite end point of CV death or first hospitalization for heart failure. The patients who were randomized into EMPEROR-Preserved were as expected based on the inclusion criteria and the population with HFPEF. Around half of the patients had type 2 diabetes and chronic kidney disease and around one-fourth had experienced a hospitalization for heart failure within the past year. The mean ejection fraction was 54%. The authors reported that there was a significant reduction of 21% in the primary comes outcome of CV death or heart hospitalizations for heart failure (HR 0.79 95%CI 0.69–0.9, $P < .001$; see **Fig. 1**) with a 29% relative risk reduction in heart failure hospitalizations (HR 0.71 95%CI 0.60–0.83) but no significant reduction in CV death (HR 0.91 95%CI 0.76–1.09; **Fig. 2**). Of the secondary end points specified in the hierarchical testing procedure, there was a significant reduction in the total number of heart failure hospitalizations (407 in the empagliflozin group vs 541 in the placebo group, a 17% relative risk reduction HR 0.73 95%CI 0.61–0.88) and kidney function slope measured by mean change in estimated glomerular filtration rate (eGFR). In other prespecified analyses, there was an improvement in the Kansas City Cardiomyopathy Questionnaire (KCCQ) clinical summary score at 52 weeks in favor of improving symptoms with empagliflozin. There was a reduction in the composite renal outcome

as a prespecified analysis, but this did not reach statistical significance neither did the reduction in the onset of new diabetes in patients with prediabetes, and there was no effect on death from any cause (HR 1.00 95%CI 0.87–1.15; see **Fig. 2**). Of the key prespecified subgroups, there was no evidence of interaction of treatment effects by diabetes at baseline or age, kidney function, body mass index, NT-proBNP, or by prior use of inhibitors of the renin angiotensin aldosterone system. Much of the prior literature of the benefit of drugs in HFREF, when examined across the ejection fraction spectrum, had demonstrated a gradient in benefit by ejection fraction with those at the higher end of the ejection fraction spectrum appearing to derive less benefit.[19–21] In EMPEROR-Preserved the point estimate for the treatment effect for the group with an ejection fraction of 60% or greater just failed to reach statistical significance. Although ordinarily this would be viewed as a subgroup analysis and not of importance given the primary outcome was met, the prior literature and similar gradients having been reported for other therapies for heart failure meant that further dissection of the relationship with ejection fraction was of interest in determining if the results were applicable to all patients with HFPEF.

EJECTION FRACTION AND EMPAGLIFLOZIN IN HEART FAILURE WITH PRESERVED EJECTION FRACTION

In a secondary analysis of the EMPEROR-Preserved trial, the effect of empagliflozin on outcomes by ejection fraction was explored.[22] There

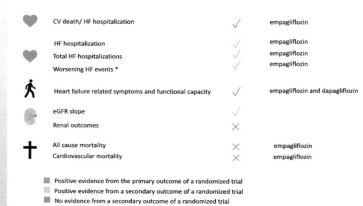

CV death/ HF hospitalization	✓	empagliflozin
HF hospitalization	✓	empagliflozin
Total HF hospitalizations	✓	empagliflozin
Worsening HF events *	✓	empagliflozin
Heart failure related symptoms and functional capacity	✓	empagliflozin and dapagliflozin
eGFR slope	✓	
Renal outcomes	✗	
All cause mortality	✗	empagliflozin
Cardiovascular mortality	✗	empagliflozin

■ Positive evidence from the primary outcome of a randomized trial
■ Positive evidence from a secondary outcome of a randomized trial
■ No evidence from a secondary outcome of a randomized trial

Fig. 2. Benefits in patients with HF with preserved ejection fraction of SGLT2 inhibitors that are currently used for the treatment of HF with reduced ejection fraction. * including emergency or urgent heart failure visit requiring intravenous treatment, requirement for intensive care or vasopressor or positive inotropic drugs and outpatient intensification of oral diuretics.

has been much debate in the literature about the point at which we define HFREF and HFPEF at the lower end of the ejection fraction spectrum. Based on secondary analyses of prior trials, there has been a move toward viewing HFREF and heart failure with mildly reduced ejection fraction as the same group in recent guidelines,[9] recognizing that patients with an ejection fraction of less than 50% tend to derive benefit from the traditionally used drugs for heart failure (angiotensin converting enzyme [ACE] inhibitors, angiotensin receptor blockers, beta blockers, and mineralocorticoid receptor antagonists). In the PARAGON-HF trial with sacubitril/valsartan an ejection fraction of around 55% seemed to similarly define those who benefited from the angiotensin receptor neprilysin inhibitor.[19] Following from this, the EMPEROR-Preserved investigators reported that when LVEF was examined as a categorical variable or as a continuous variable a very clear gradient in benefit of impact of empagliflozin with an ejection fraction below what would be called normal (<55%). Because the investigators were able to combine the EMPEROR-Preserved and EMPEROR-Reduced trials, there were enough events to examine each of the categories of ejection fraction to define where a cut off in benefit may lie. They found that above and ejection fraction of 65%, there was attenuation of the benefit of empagliflozin, although overall there was no evidence of heterogeneity in the treatment effect by ejection fraction (P value for interaction equal to 0.3). They also examined the interaction with sex as an analysis of the PARAGON-HF trial suggested that there was an interaction with sex that may have been in part explained by different ejection fraction thresholds for normal in men and women.[23] The EMPEROR-Preserved investigators did not find a treatment by sex by LVEF interaction. Although these are interesting data and confirm the findings of other recent analyses in

HFPEF with other drugs, they are exploratory in nature and the results of the primary analysis of EMPEROR-Preserved stand, empagliflozin reduced the risk of CV death or heart failure hospitalization in patients with heart failure and an ejection fraction of greater than 40%.

HEART FAILURE OUTCOMES

As may be expected from the primary results of EMPEROR-Preserved, there are several analyses that support using the SGLT2 inhibitor empagliflozin to reduce the risk of worsening heart failure outcomes. A broad range of outcomes related to heart failure was recorded in EMPEROR-Preserved (see **Fig. 2**). These included heart failure hospitalizations, total HF hospitalizations, requirement for intravenous vasopressor or inotropic support, admission to intensive care unit, requirement for urgent care/emergency department visits and outpatient intravenous diuretic therapy.[24] For all of these outcomes, and for multiple composite outcomes composed of these different heart failure-related outcomes, there was a clear reduction in the risk of each with empagliflozin in patients with HFPEF. Only the reduction in total hospitalizations for any reason was not statistically significantly reduced in the empagliflozin group.

HEART FAILURE-RELATED QUALITY OF LIFE AND FUNCTIONAL CAPACITY

Patients with HFPEF are characterized by marked limitation in physical functioning and a high burden of heart failure-related symptoms. Therefore, improving heart failure-related health status (symptoms, functional status, and quality of life) is a key aim of the treatment of HFPEF. One of the key prespecified secondary end points in EMPEROR-Preserved was improvement in a self-reported measure of heart failure-related symptoms, function, and quality of life, measured by the KCCQ.[18] The domain used in the prespecified secondary analysis was the total symptom score. This was improved by empagliflozin, and in further analyses, both the clinical summary score and overall summary score were also improved.[25] There was also a clear increase in the proportion of patients reporting an improvement of 5 points, 10 points, and 15 points in the patients randomized to empagliflozin and, conversely, a reduction in the number of patients reporting a deterioration by 5 points or more. Importantly, there is no evidence that the benefit of empagliflozin differed by baseline KCCQ score. These results were in contrast to the EMPERIAL trial,[26,27] which examined if empagliflozin improved 6 minute walk distance in 315 patients with an LVEF greater than 40%. They did not find any effect of empagliflozin on 6 minute walk distance (median difference between placebo and empagliflozin of 4.0 m [−5.0, 13.0; P = .37]). Another trial, PRESERVED-HF[28] did however report an improvement in 6 minute walk test distance with dapagliflozin in 324 patients with and LVEF 45% or greater as well as replicating the benefits on KCCQ scores seen with empagliflozin in EMPEROR-Preserved (see **Fig. 2**).

KIDNEY OUTCOMES

There is ample evidence from prior trials of SGLT2 inhibitors that they preserve kidney function and reduce the risk of kidney outcomes.[4,29] Because chronic kidney disease is a common comorbidity in HFPEF, any effect of SGLT2i on kidney outcomes would be beneficial. In a prespecified secondary outcome in the hierarchical testing of the EMPEROR-Preserved trial, the reduction in the slope of eGFR was statistically significant in favor of empagliflozin.[18] This was similar to the findings in HFREF with dapagliflozin and empagliflozin.[30,31] However, slowing of decline in eGFR may not always mirror the effect on kidney outcomes and is not a perfect surrogate measure. There was no reduction in endpoint of the combined kidney outcomes in EMPEROR-Preserved in contrast to EMPEROR-Reduced and a meta-analysis of EMPEROR-Reduced and DAPA-HF.[32] In a prespecified pooled analysis of EMPEROR-Preserved and EMPEROR-Reduced there was a statistically significant interaction between trial and randomized therapy on kidney outcomes (profound and sustained decreases in eGFR or renal-replacement therapy).[33] The HRs were 0.51 (95% CI 0.33–0.79) in the EMPEROR-Reduced trial and 0.95 (95% CI 0.73–1.24) in the EMPEROR-Preserved trial (P = .016 for interaction). Therefore,

whether SGLT2 inhibitors improve kidney outcomes in HFPEF is still unknown.

POTENTIAL MECHANISMS OF BENEFIT OF SGLT2i IN HEART FAILURE WITH PRESERVED EJECTION FRACTION

As described above, SGLT2 inhibitors improve morbidity and mortality in HFPEF, improve heart failure-related symptoms and improve functional capacity and slow the deterioration in kidney function. There is much speculation about the proposed mechanism of action of SGLT2 inhibitors [34] and several studies are being conducted to try and illuminate a particular pathway.[35] In HFREF, one mechanism that has been demonstrated is improvement in left ventricular (LV) size.[36] This is not likely to be the same in HFPEF where cardiac structure and function is different. However, in most trials of pharmacotherapy in HFPEF, there is a requirement of some structural heart disease to be present (either left atrial enlargement or left ventricular hypertrophy) because these are thought to be hallmarks of the disease. It is possible that these 2 parameters may be improved by SGLT2i, with experimental evidence suggesting that SGLT2i improves cardiac hypertrophy and diastolic function,[37,38] and evidence that alterations in myocardial energy utilization may be the other important factor.[39,40] Another potential mechanism is the general improvement in kidney function. This has already been shown in patients with HFREF, and the benefits of SGLT2i are also evident in those with chronic kidney disease; therefore, a kidney benefit may translate into improved HF status, particularly in HFPEF where renal dysfunction is common.

FUTURE TRIALS OF SGLT2 INHIBITORS IN HEART FAILURE WITH PRESERVED EJECTION FRACTION

Although the EMPEROR-Preserved results were a landmark for the treatment of HFPEF, being only one trial, which did not show any benefit on mortality, the results of other trials of SGLT2 inhibitors in HFPEF are keenly awaited. The DELIVER trial randomized 6263 patients with a left ventricular ejection fraction of more than 40% with elevated natriuretic peptides (≥300 pg/mL if in sinus rhythm or ≥600 pg/mL if in atrial fibrillation/flutter) and evidence of structural heart disease (left atrial [LA] enlargement or LV hypertrophy) to dapagliflozin 10 mg/d or placebo on top of usual medication according to regional standard of care.[41] The primary composite of worsening heart failure episodes (either unplanned hospitalization or urgent heart failure visit requiring intravenous therapy but not requiring a hospital admission) or CV death will be analyzed as time-to-first event. However, given the information gained from PARAGON-HF, and now EMPEROR-Preserved, the end point will be assessed in a dual primary analysis in the full study population and those with and ejection fraction of less than 60%.

The results of the DELIVER trial are keenly anticipated to see if they confirm the results of EMPEROR-Preserved. Furthermore, there is interest in whether DELIVER will demonstrate a benefit of a SGLT2i in reducing mortality in HFPEF, which was not seen in EMPEROR-Preserved. There is hope that this might be plausible given that dapagliflozin reduced mortality in DAPA-HF but empagliflozin did not in EMPEROR-Reduced and meta-analysis of the 2 trials confirmed the mortality reduction with SGLT2 inhibitors in HFREF,[32] we can hope for the same in HFPEF. However, from the analyses of EMPEROR-Preserved described, the European Medicines Agency Committee for Medicinal Products for Human Use adopted a positive opinion recommending a change to the terms of the marketing authorization for empagliflozin.[42] The indication will be changed from "…adults for the treatment of symptomatic chronic heart failure with reduced ejection fraction" to "…adults for the treatment of symptomatic chronic heart failure" thereby removing the ejection fraction requirement and opening up the therapy to patients with HFPEF. How this new indication is incorporated into guidelines remains to be resolved. Given the lack of any disease-modifying drugs for HFPEF in the guidelines, it is likely that empagliflozin will be the initial therapy of choice for HFPEF and may also be joined by dapagliflozin dependent on the results of DELIVER should a class effect be observed.

SUMMARY

Patients with HFPEF now join patients with type 2 diabetes, HFREF and patients with chronic kidney disease (CKD) as a group who can derive benefit from the SGLT2 inhibitors. After many failures, in empagliflozin, we finally have a therapy for HFPEF that can alter the prognosis of patients as well as improve heart failure-related symptoms. This is a major step forward in the treatment of HFPEF and will undoubtedly shape future guidelines on the management of heart failure.

DISCLOSURE

P.S. Jhund's employer has been remunerated by AstraZeneca, Bayer, Novartis, and NovoNordisk for work on clinical trials. P.S. Jhund has received speaker fees and advisory board fees from AstraZeneca, Boehringer Ingelheim, and Novartis and research funding from Boehringer Ingelheim and Analog Devices Inc.

REFERENCES

1. Zinman B, Wanner C, Lachin JM, et al. Empagliflozin, cardiovascular outcomes, and mortality in type 2 diabetes. N Engl J Med 2015;373:2117–28.
2. Wiviott SD, Raz I, Bonaca MP, et al. Dapagliflozin and cardiovascular outcomes in type 2 diabetes. N Engl J Med 2019;380:347–57.
3. Neal B, Perkovic V, Mahaffey KW, et al. Canagliflozin and cardiovascular and renal events in type 2 diabetes. N Engl J Med 2017;377:644–57.
4. Perkovic V, Jardine MJ, Neal B, et al. Canagliflozin and renal outcomes in type 2 diabetes and nephropathy. N Engl J Med 2019;380:2295–306.
5. Cannon CP, Pratley R, Dagogo-Jack S, et al. Cardiovascular outcomes with ertugliflozin in type 2 diabetes. N Engl J Med 2020;383:1425–35.
6. McMurray JJV, Solomon SD, Inzucchi SE, et al. Dapagliflozin in patients with heart failure and reduced ejection fraction. N Engl J Med 2019;381:1995–2008.
7. Packer M, Anker SD, Butler J, et al. Cardiovascular and renal outcomes with empagliflozin in heart failure. N Engl J Med 2020;383:1413–24. NEJMoa2022190.
8. Dunlay SM, Roger VL, Redfield MM. Epidemiology of heart failure with preserved ejection fraction. Nat Rev Cardiol 2017;14:591–602.
9. Authors/Task Force Members, McDonagh TA, Metra M, Adamo M, et al. 2021 ESC Guidelines for the diagnosis and treatment of acute and chronic heart failure: Developed by the Task Force for the diagnosis and treatment of acute and chronic heart failure of the European Society of Cardiology (ESC). With the special contribution of the Heart Failure Association (HFA) of the ESC. Eur J Heart Fail 2022;24:4–131.
10. Fitchett D, Zinman B, Wanner C, et al. Heart failure outcomes with empagliflozin in patients with type 2 diabetes at high cardiovascular risk: results of the EMPA-REG OUTCOME® trial. Eur Heart J 2016;37:1526–34.
11. Kato ET, Silverman MG, Mosenzon O, et al. Effect of dapagliflozin on heart failure and mortality in type 2 diabetes mellitus. Circulation 2019;139:2528–36.
12. Berg DD, Jhund PS, Docherty KF, et al. Time to clinical benefit of dapagliflozin and significance of prior heart failure hospitalization in patients with heart failure with reduced ejection fraction. JAMA Cardiol 2021. https://doi.org/10.1001/jamacardio.2020.7585.
13. Bhatt DL, Szarek M, Steg PG, et al. Sotagliflozin in patients with diabetes and recent worsening heart failure. N Engl J Med 2020;384:117–28.

14. Bhatt DL, Szarek M, Pitt B, et al. Sotagliflozin in Patients with Diabetes and Chronic Kidney Disease. N Engl J Med 2021;384:129–39.

15. Bhatt DL, et al. American College of Cardiology Virtual Annual Scientific Session (ACC 2021). 2021. Available at: https://www.acc.org/latest-in-cardiology/clinical-trials/2020/11/11/22/00/soloist-whf. Accessed February 10, 2022.

16. Solomon SD, McMurray JJV, Anand IS, et al. Angiotensin-neprilysin inhibition in heart failure with preserved ejection fraction. N Engl J Med 2019;381:1609–20.

17. Anker SD, Butler J, Filippatos GS, et al. Evaluation of the effects of sodium–glucose co-transporter 2 inhibition with empagliflozin on morbidity and mortality in patients with chronic heart failure and a preserved ejection fraction: rationale for and design of the EMPEROR-Preserved Trial. Eur J Heart Fail 2019;21:1279–87.

18. Anker SD, Butler J, Filippatos G, et al. Empagliflozin in Heart Failure with a Preserved Ejection Fraction. N Engl J Med 2021;385:1451–61.

19. Solomon SD, Vaduganathan M, Claggett BL, et al. Sacubitril/valsartan across the spectrum of ejection fraction in heart failure. Circulation 2020;141:352–61.

20. Lund LH, Claggett B, Liu J, et al. Heart failure with mid-range ejection fraction in CHARM: characteristics, outcomes and effect of candesartan across the entire ejection fraction spectrum. Eur J Heart Fail 2018;20:1230–9.

21. Abdul-Rahim AH, Shen L, Rush CJ, et al. Effect of digoxin in patients with heart failure and mid-range (borderline) left ventricular ejection fraction. Eur J Heart Fail 2018;20:1139–45.

22. Butler J, Packer M, Filippatos G, et al. Effect of empagliflozin in patients with heart failure across the spectrum of left ventricular ejection fraction. Eur Heart J 2022;43:416–26.

23. McMurray JJV, Jackson AM, Lam CSP, et al. Effects of sacubitril-valsartan versus valsartan in women compared with men with heart failure and preserved ejection fraction: insights from PARAGON-HF. Circulation 2020. https://doi.org/10.1161/CIRCULATIONAHA.119.044491.

24. Packer M, Butler J, Zannad F, et al. Effect of empagliflozin on worsening heart failure events in patients with heart failure and preserved ejection fraction: EMPEROR-preserved trial. Circulation 2021;144:1284–94.

25. Butler J, Filippatos G, Jamal Siddiqi T, et al. Empagliflozin, health status, and quality of life in patients with heart failure and preserved ejection fraction: The EMPEROR-Preserved Trial. Circulation 2022;145:184–93.

26. Abraham WT, Ponikowski P, Brueckmann M, et al. Rationale and design of the EMPERIAL-preserved and EMPERIAL-reduced trials of empagliflozin in patients with chronic heart failure. Eur J Heart Fail 2019;21:932–42.

27. Abraham WT, Lindenfeld JA, Ponikowski P, et al. Effect of empagliflozin on exercise ability and symptoms in heart failure patients with reduced and preserved ejection fraction, with and without type 2 diabetes. Eur Heart J 2021;42:700–10.

28. Nassif ME, Windsor SL, Borlaug BA, et al. The SGLT2 inhibitor dapagliflozin in heart failure with preserved ejection fraction: a multicenter randomized trial. Nat Med 2021;27(11):1954–60.

29. Heerspink HJL, Stefánsson BV, Correa-Rotter R, et al. Dapagliflozin in Patients with Chronic Kidney Disease. N Engl J Med 2020;383:1436–46.

30. Jhund PS, Solomon SD, Docherty KF, et al. Efficacy of dapagliflozin on renal function and outcomes in patients with heart failure with reduced ejection fraction: results of DAPA-HF. Circulation 2021;143:298–309.

31. Zannad F, Ferreira JP, Pocock SJ, et al. Cardiac and kidney benefits of empagliflozin in heart failure across the spectrum of kidney function: insights from EMPEROR-reduced. Circulation 2021;143:310–21.

32. Zannad F, Ferreira JP, Pocock SJ, et al. SGLT2 inhibitors in patients with heart failure with reduced ejection fraction: a meta-analysis of the EMPEROR-Reduced and DAPA-HF trials. Lancet 2020;396:819–29.

33. Packer M, Butler J, Zannad F, et al. Empagliflozin and major renal outcomes in heart failure. N Engl J Med 2021;385:1531–3.

34. Lopaschuk GD, Verma S. Mechanisms of cardiovascular benefits of sodium glucose Co-Transporter 2 (SGLT2) inhibitors: a state-of-the-art review. JACC Basic Transl Sci 2020;5:632–44.

35. Lee MMY, Petrie MC, McMurray JJV, et al. How Do SGLT2 (Sodium-Glucose Cotransporter 2) Inhibitors and GLP-1 (Glucagon-Like Peptide-1) Receptor Agonists Reduce Cardiovascular Outcomes?: Completed and Ongoing Mechanistic Trials. Arterioscler Thromb Vasc Biol 2020;40:506–22.

36. Lee MMY, Brooksbank KJM, Wetherall K, et al. Effect of Empagliflozin on Left Ventricular Volumes in Patients with Type 2 Diabetes, or Prediabetes, and Heart Failure with Reduced Ejection Fraction (SUGAR-DM-HF). Circulation 2021;143:516–25.

37. Verma S, Mazer CD, Yan AT, et al. Effect of empagliflozin on left ventricular mass in patients with Type 2 diabetes and coronary artery disease: The EMPA-HEART CardioLink-6 randomized clinical trial. Circulation 2019;140(21):1693–702.

38. Connelly KA, Zhang Y, Visram A, et al. Empagliflozin Improves Diastolic Function in a Nondiabetic Rodent Model of Heart Failure With Preserved Ejection Fraction. JACC Basic Transl Sci 2019;4:27–37.

39. Ferrannini E, Muscelli E, Frascerra S, et al. Metabolic response to sodium-glucose cotransporter 2 inhibition in type 2 diabetic patients. J Clin Invest 2014; 124:499–508.

40. Ferrannini E, Baldi S, Frascerra S, et al. Shift to fatty substrate utilization in response to sodium-glucose cotransporter 2 inhibition in subjects without diabetes and patients with type 2 diabetes. Diabetes 2016;65:1190–5.

41. Solomon SD, Boer RA, DeMets D, et al. Dapagliflozin in heart failure with preserved and mildly reduced ejection fraction: rationale and design of the DELIVER trial. Eur J Heart Fail 2021;23:1217–25.

42. Available at: https://www.ema.europa.eu/en/medicines/human/summaries-opinion/jardiance-0. Accessed February 10, 2022.

SGLT2 Inhibitors in Heart Failure
Early Initiation to Achieve Rapid Clinical Benefits

Neal M. Dixit, MD, MBA[a], Boback Ziaeian, MD, PhD[a,b,c],
Gregg C. Fonarow, MD[a,b,*]

KEYWORDS

- Heart failure with reduced ejection fraction • Heart failure with preserved ejection fraction
- Initiation and sequencing • Guideline-directed medical therapy

KEY POINTS

- SGLT2i are high-value medications that demonstrate morbidity and mortality benefits within 30 days of initiation.
- SGLT2i should be initiated simultaneously or in rapid sequence with the other core pillars of GDMT before device therapy consideration.
- In-hospital initiation of SGLT2i is well tolerated and safe and reduces the risk of rehospitalization and death.
- SGLT2i reduce heart failure (HF) hospitalization in HF patients with EF greater than 40% and are a valuable potential therapy in a population with few therapeutic options.

INTRODUCTION

More than 60 million people are living with heart failure (HF) worldwide and as many as one-third may die within the next year.[1,2] Immense progress has been made in the discovery of life-saving medications for patients with HF. However, these therapies are persistently underused.[3] The recent addition of sodium-glucose cotransporter-2 inhibitors (SGLT2i), in addition to standard therapies for HF with reduced ejection fraction (HFrEF), has made them the newest class (**Fig. 1**) of guideline-directed medical therapies (GDMTs).[4] SGLT2i also demonstrate clinical benefits in HF with moderately reduced ejection fraction/ heart failure with preserved ejection fraction (HFmrEF/ HFpEF),[5] diabetes,[6] and chronic kidney disease (CKD).[7]

In a meta-analysis of the SGLT2i randomized controlled trials (RCTs) for HFrEF, treatment with dapagliflozin and empagliflozin, resulted in a 13% reduction in all-cause mortality and a 25% reduction in cardiovascular hospitalization versus placebo.[8] These benefits were seen as soon as 12 days after initiation.[9,10] Although no formal guidelines have been published regarding the optimal timing of initiation of SGLT2i in HFrEF, the clinical benefits of SGLT2i warrant simultaneous or rapid initiation alongside the other pillars of GDMT at the time of diagnosis (**Fig. 2**). We will provide an overview of the benefits of SGLT2i, concomitant initiation alongside other GDMT medications, hospital initiation, cost and value considerations, and benefits in patients with HFmrEF and HFpEF.

[a] Department of Medicine, David Geffen School of Medicine at UCLA, Los Angeles, CA, USA; [b] Division of Cardiology, David Geffen School of Medicine at UCLA, Los Angeles, CA, USA; [c] Division of Cardiology, Veteran Affairs Greater Los Angeles Healthcare System, Los Angeles, CA, USA
* Corresponding author. A2-237 CHS, Mail Code: 167917650 Charles E Young Dr. S, Los Angeles, CA 90095-1679.
E-mail address: gfonarow@mednet.ucla.edu
Twitter: @NealDixit (N.M.D.); @boback (B.Z.); @gcfmd (G.C.F.)

Heart Failure Clin 18 (2022) 587–596
https://doi.org/10.1016/j.hfc.2022.03.003
1551-7136/22/© 2022 Elsevier Inc. All rights reserved.

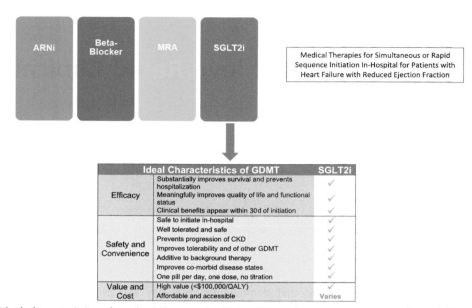

Fig. 1. Ideal characteristics of medical therapy for HF. ARNi, angiotensin receptor-neprilysin inhibitors; CKD, chronic kidney disease; GDMT, guideline-directed medical therapy; HFrEF, heart failure with reduced ejection fraction; MRA, mineralocorticoid-receptor antagonists; QALY, quality-adjusted life year; SGLT2i, sodium-glucose cotransporter-2 inhibitors.

THE NEAR-IMMEDIATE BENEFIT OF SGLT2i

Before the emergence of SGLT2i, consensus GDMT for HFrEF included beta-blockers (BBs), renin–angiotensin–aldosterone system inhibitors (RAASi)/angiotensin receptor-neprilysin inhibitors (ARNis), and mineralocorticoid-receptor antagonists (MRAs), all of which reduce mortality, morbidity, and have onset of clinical benefit within 30 days of initiation.[11] SGLT2i have likewise demonstrated this near-immediate benefit in RCTs, demonstrating improvement in cardiovascular outcomes within 30 days with dapagliflozin and empagliflozin (**Table 1**).

In analysis of the dapagliflozin in patients with HF and reduced ejection fraction (DAPA-HF) trial, the primary outcome of worsening HF event or cardiovascular death reached statistical significance in favor of the dapagliflozin arm at just 28 days and remained significant for the remainder of the trial.[12] Similarly, in the Empagliflozin Outcome Trial in Patients With Chronic Heart Failure and a Reduced Ejection Fraction (EMPEROR-Reduced) trial, empagliflozin achieved statistical significance for the primary outcome of worsening HF event or death by day 12.[9] Several possible mechanisms of cardiovascular benefit derived

Initial Visit or Hospitalization	Follow-up →			Clinical Benefits			
Days 1–4	Days 7–14	Days 14–28	Days 28–56	RRR of All-Cause Mortality in Meta-analysis	RRR of HF Hospitalization in Meta-analysis	Clinical Benefits within 30d of Initiation Demonstrate?	In-Hospital Initiation Safe and Well Tolerated?
ARNi		Continue	Titrate, as tolerated	Titrate, as tolerated	28%[a]	49%[a]	✓	✓
Beta-Blocker	Titrate, as tolerated	Titrate, as tolerated	Titrate, as tolerated	31%	37%	✓	✓
MRA		Continue	Titrate, as tolerated	Continue	25%	23%	✓	✓
SGLT2i		Continue	Continue	Continue	13%	25%	✓	✓

Fig. 2. Suggested method of simultaneous or rapid-sequence initiation of quadruple medical therapy for HFrEF with associated clinical benefits. ARNi, angiotensin receptor-neprilysin inhibitors; HF, heart failure; HFrEF, heart failure with reduced ejection fraction; MRA, mineralocorticoid-receptor antagonists; RRR, relative risk reduction; SGLT2i, sodium-glucose cotransporter-2 inhibitors. [a] Computed versus putative placebo in analysis of PARADIGM-HF Trial.

Table 1
Summary of clinical benefits of SGLT2i in clinical trials

Trial	Sample Size (n)	Intervention	Inclusion Criteria	Setting	Primary Outcome	Overall Treatment Effect (95% CI)	Time to Significant Benefit (days)	AE Leading to Discontinuation (Drug vs Placebo)
DAPA-HF	4744	Dapagliflozin 10 mg O.D. vs placebo	LVEF ≤40%; NYHA II–IV; eGFR ≥30 mL/ min/1.73 m²	Outpatient	Worsening HF or CV death	HR = 0.74 (0.65– 0.85)	28	4.7% vs 4.9%
EMPEROR-Reduced	3730	Empagliflozin 10 mg O.D. vs placebo	LVEF ≤40%; NYHA II–IV; eGFR ≥20 mL/ min/1.73 m²	Outpatient	HF hospitalization or CV death	HR = 0.75 (0.65– 0.86)	12[a]	8.5% vs 8.9%
EMPA-RESPONSE-AHF	79	Empagliflozin 10 mg O.D. vs placebo	Hospitalized for acute HF; eGFR ≥ 30 mL/min/ 1.73 m²	Inpatient	Change in dyspnea, diuretic response, length of initial hospital stay, and change in NT-proBNP	NS	–	17.5% vs 12.8%
SOLOIST-WHF	1222	Sotagliflozin 200 mg O.D. vs placebo	Type-2 diabetes; recent worsening HF; eGFR ≥30 mL/ min/1.73 m²	48.8% initiated inpatient and 51.2% early after discharge	Total number of CV deaths and hospitalizations and urgent HF visits	HR = 0.67 (0.52– 0.85)	28	7.8% vs 6.6%
EMPEROR-Preserved	5988	Empagliflozin 10 mg O.D. vs placebo	LVEF >40%; NYHA II–IV; eGFR ≥20 mL/min/ 1.73 m²	Outpatient	HF hospitalization or CV death	HR = 0.79 (0.69– 0.90)	18	19.1% vs 18.4%

(continued on next page)

Table 1
(continued)

Trial	Sample Size (n)	Intervention	Inclusion Criteria	Setting	Primary Outcome	Overall Treatment Effect (95% CI)	Time to Significant Benefit (days)	AE Leading to Discontinuation (Drug vs Placebo)
EMPULSE	530	Empagliflozin 10 mg O.D. vs placebo	Hospitalized for acute HF; eGFR ≥ 30 mL/min/1.73 m²	Inpatient	Win ratio (composite of death, HF events, and change in KCCQ-TSS)	Win ratio = 1.36 (1.09–1.68)	90[b]	NR

Abbreviations: AE, adverse event; CI, confidence interval; CV, cardiovascular; DAPA-HF, dapagliflozin and prevention of adverse outcome in heart failure; eGFR, estimated glomerular filtration rate; EMPA-RESPONSE-AHF, randomized, Double-Blind, Placebo-Controlled, Multicenter Pilot Study On The Effects Of Empagliflozin On Clinical Outcomes In Patients With Acute Decompensated Heart Failure; EMPEROR-Preserved, Empagliflozin Outcome Trial In Patients With Chronic Heart Failure With Preserved Ejection Fraction; EMPEROR-Reduced, Empagliflozin Outcome Trial in Patients with Chronic Heart Failure and a Reduced Ejection Fraction; EMPULSE, A Study to Test the Effect of Empagliflozin in Patients Who Are in Hospital for Acute Heart Failure; HF, heart failure; KCCQ-TSS, Kansas City Cardiomyopathy Questionnaires total summary score; LVEF, left ventricular ejection fraction; NR, not reported; NS, non-significant; NT-proBNP, N-terminal (NT)-prohormone BNP; NYHA, New York Heart Association; O.D., once a day; SGLT2i, sodium-glucose cotransporter 2 inhibitor; SOLOIST-WHF, Effect of Sotagliflozin on Cardiovascular Events in Patients with Type 2 Diabetes Post Worsening Heart Failure

[a] Statistical significance was first reached at 12 d but was sustained from day 34.
[b] Analysis at a time point before 90 not currently available.

from SGLT2i have been identified.[13] A few mechanisms that have been shown to occur early and may be the basis for the observed clinical benefits are outlined.

Reverse Ventricular Remodeling

Pathologic cardiac remodeling associated with HFrEF increases the risk for hospitalization and death by increasing the likelihood of volume overload, pump failure, or ventricular arrhythmia.[14] Reverse ventricular remodeling is observed with BB, RAASi/ARNi, and MRA usage.[15] The impact of SGLT2i on reverse ventricular remodeling was studied in the Randomized Trial of Empagliflozin in Nondiabetic Patients With Heart Failure and Reduced Ejection Fraction (EMPA-TROPISM) trial.[16] In the 6-month trial period, the empagliflozin arm (compared with placebo) had large improvements in left ventricle (LV) end-diastolic volume (−25.1 vs −1.5 mL, $P < .001$), LV end-systolic volume (−26.6 vs −0.5 mL, $P < .001$), LV mass (−17.8 vs 4.1 g, $P < .001$), and LV sphericity. Left ventricular ejection fraction (LVEF) was also improved (6.0 vs −0.1, $P < .001$).

Although the change in LV architecture was assessed at 6 months, the magnitude of the effect combined with known early clinical benefits of SGLT2i implies that these changes are likely occurring soon after initiation. The mechanism for the rapid reverse remodeling was speculated by the same group to be due to, in part, to SGLT2i induced switching of myocardial energy consumption from glucose to fatty acids, ketone bodies, and branched-chain amino acids.[17] However, further research to elucidate the complete mechanism of SGLT2i-induced reverse ventricular remodeling is needed.

Decongestion Without Neurohormonal Compensation

Initiation of SGLT2i has been shown to cause diuresis and natriuresis without the compensatory neurohormonal activation that results from diuresis with traditional diuretics.[18] In the Randomized, double-blind, placebo-controlled, multicenter pilot study on the effects of empagliflozin on clinical outcomes in patients with acute decompensated heart failure (EMPA-RESPONSE-AHF) trial, hospitalized patients with HFrEF were initiated on empagliflozin or placebo.[19] Although the trial showed no significant differences in the primary endpoints (change in dyspnea, diuretic response, length of stay, and N-terminal probrain natriuretic peptide level), the data reported in the exploratory outcomes suggests increased net urine output (∼850 mL/d) in the empagliflozin group compared with the placebo group during the first 4 days of hospitalization.

Similarly, a single-center crossover placebo-controlled trial of stable HFrEF patients with diabetes showed that empagliflozin significantly increased fractional excretion of sodium with a resultant 138 mL ($P = .04$) reduction in plasma volume at 14 days compared with placebo.[20] Interestingly, plasma norepinephrine levels measured at 14 days increased only 0.09 nmol/L in the empagliflozin group compared with 0.7 nmol/L in the placebo group ($P = .023$). There was no difference in levels of other neurohormones (renin, aldosterone, copeptin).

These two studies suggest that SGLT2i induce a greater reduction in plasma volume by way of increased diuresis and natriuresis without the increase in compensatory neurohormonal activation that precedes ventricular remodeling.[21]

Increase in Erythropoietin

In a substudy of the Effects of Empagliflozin on Cardiac Structure in Patients With Type 2 Diabetes (EMPA-HEART) trial, investigators measured erythropoietin levels at 0, 1, and 6 months after initiation of empagliflozin.[22] At just 1 month, erythropoietin levels were significantly increased in the empagliflozin arm (compared with placebo). Additionally, hematocrit level was found to be significantly increased by 6 months in the empagliflozin arm. Hematocrit was similarly increased in the Empagliflozin in Heart Failure with a Preserved Ejection Fraction (EMPEROR-Preserved) trial at just 1 month. Erythropoietin has previously been shown to have systemic cardioprotective effects[23] in addition to reducing the likelihood of anemia, a known risk factor of HF morbidity and mortality.[22,24] In patients with HFrEF, improvements in erythropoietin and hematocrit levels may be an additional early protective mechanism of SGLT2i.

INITIATION OF SGLT2i WITH OR WITHOUT BACKGROUND THERAPY

The most effective method to maximize relative risk reduction of HF hospitalization and all-cause mortality is simultaneous or rapid sequence initiation of all four pillars of GDMT.[25] Traditional sequencing methods, aiming to maximize BB and RAASi dosage before MRA or SGLT2i initiation, result in unnecessary delays in the initiation of crucial GDMT agents. In fact, the effectiveness of SGLT2i is not dependent on the presence or absence of background HFrEF therapy, and they are well tolerated (and even act synergistically) with other GDMT agents.

In Docherty and colleagues's analysis of the DAPA-HF trial, there was a consistent benefit of dapagliflozin over placebo regardless of whether patients were optimized on guideline-recommended doses, only partially optimized, or were not on GDMT at all.[26] Additionally, in the Empagliflozin in Patients Hospitalized for Acute Heart Failure (EMPULSE) trial, 33% of patients presented with *de novo* HF and were not yet on GDMT, but SGLT2i still demonstrated a magnitude of the effect similar to DAPA-HF and EMPEROR-Reduced.[27]

Importantly, SGLT2i may increase tolerance for other GDMT agents. In both the DAPA-HF and EMPEROR-Reduced trials, patients on MRA that were randomized to treatment with SGLT2i were less likely to experience hyperkalemia.[28,29] In turn, this may be a contributing reason for why patients on SGLT2i have less discontinuation of MRA for which hyperkalemia is a common side effect and reason for discontinuation.[29] The mechanism of MRA tolerance is not known.

Moreover, SGLT2i are consistently associated with reduced adverse kidney outcomes and slow the progression of CKD.[30,31] Therefore, the renoprotective benefits of SGLT2i will likely result in fewer patients discontinuing RAASi/ARNi therapy due to reductions in glomerular filtration rate (GFR).[31]

Although benefits to BB tolerance have not been shown, SGLT2i have minimal blood pressure effect in patients with low blood pressure and are unlikely to result in intolerance to BB due to hypotension. In hypertensive patients, SGLT2i can act as effective antihypertensives, exhibiting a reduction in systolic blood pressure (SBP) of ~3 to 9 mm Hg versus placebo in several trials.[32] However, in a subgroup analysis of patients with an SBP less than 110 mm Hg in the EMPEROR-Reduced trial, no blood pressure difference was seen during the duration of the trial in the empagliflozin group versus placebo group.[33] Similar findings in the SBP less than 110 mm Hg group were seen in the analysis of the DAPA-HF trial.[34] In both trials, the effect size of SGLT2i on the primary outcomes was consistent across all SBP levels.[33,34]

To date, no pillar of GDMT has demonstrated any diminishment of effect by the presence of any combination of background therapy.[35] SGLT2i continue this trend, demonstrating additive the benefit that may actually enable tolerance for additional therapy. Additionally, due to the minimal adverse effects, the initiation of SGLT2i is unlikely to limit efforts to initiate and titrate the other pillars of GDMT.

SGLT2i BEFORE DEVICE THERAPY

Implantable cardiac defibrillators (ICDs), cardiac resynchronization therapy (CRT), and transcatheter edge-edge mitral valve repair (TEER) are three therapies with a demonstrated mortality benefit in eligible populations with HFrEF.[4] To ensure the maximal benefit and demonstrate medical necessity, guidelines recommend, with all three therapies, that patients be initiated on GDMT (and typically up-titrated during a period $\geq$3 months) before consideration for intervention.[4,36] Although SGLT2i were not a pillar of core GDMT at the time of the landmark trials for these interventions, it is logical as the standard of GDMT evolves to ensure the initiation of SGLT2i before these invasive procedures. Especially, as the benefits of SGLT2i can be achieved rapidly, at a single dosage, and may induce reverse cardiac remodeling of the heart to such a degree that the device therapy is no longer required. For example, in the EMPA-TROPISM trial, LVEF increased by 6% points over the 6-month trial period.[16] This change would push many patients above the 35% LVEF threshold for ICD or CRT consideration. Additionally, although no trial has specifically evaluated improvement in secondary mitral regurgitation (MR) with SGLT2i, we can assume that SGLT2i are likely to have a beneficial effect on secondary MR due to the significant reverse cardiac remodeling effect seen in EMPA-TROPISM.[17] Thus, many patients with secondary MR after initiation of SGLT2i may no longer qualify for TEER, which requires, at least moderate-severe MR on optimal GDMT before intervention.[36]

SHOULD SGLT2i BE INITIATED DURING HOSPITALIZATION?

Despite advances in GDMT and targeted health policy, readmission and mortality rates within 30 days of HF hospitalization have not substantially declined.[37,38] A major contributing factor is exceedingly frequent deferral of initiation and titration of GDMT for HFrEF in both inpatient and outpatient settings.[3] Patients discharged from the hospital without a core pillar of GDMT have a >75% of not being started on that medication in the following year.[35] Thus, given the strong clinical inertia in the outpatient setting and the rapid benefits of all four pillars of GDMT (see **Table 1**), in-hospital initiation of core GDMT has massive potential to reduce HF hospitalization and mortality.

Although SGLT2i were initiated in the outpatient setting in the landmark DAPA-HF and EMPEROR-Reduced trials,[10,39] there is no evidence to suggest that in-hospital initiation is unsafe. On the contrary, ample evidence exists that support the notion for in-hospital initiation of SGLT2i. In the EMPA-RESPONSE-AHF trial, empagliflozin was initiated in stable hospitalized HFrEF patients and continued for 30 days.[19] As previously mentioned, the study did not meet its primary outcomes, but all safety outcomes were met, with no difference in adverse events or drug discontinuation with the empagliflozin group compared with placebo. In the SOLOIST-WHF (Effect of Sotagliflozin on Cardiovascular Events in Patients With Type 2 Diabetes Post Worsening Heart Failure) trial, the dual SGLT1/SGLT2 inhibitor, sotagliflozin, reduced the primary endpoint of cardiovascular mortality or HF hospitalization/urgent care visit by 33% versus placebo in patients with HF and diabetes.[40] In the trial, sotagliflozin was initiated before or shortly after hospital discharge, and there was no heterogeneity in efficacy between the subgroups started in-hospital or shortly after hospital discharge. Benefits were seen in the first 28 days from initiation. Serious adverse events led to a discontinuation rate in the sotagliflozin group of only 3.0% (vs 2.8% in the placebo group). Most recently, the EMPULSE trial demonstrated the safety rapid clinical benefits in hemodynamically stable HF patients initiated on SGLT2i early during hospitalizations for acute HF.[27] Patients initiated on empagliflozin were 36% more likely to receive clinical benefit than those initiated on placebo during the 3-month study period. Significant improvement in symptoms was noted at just 15 days. No safety concerns were identified, and there was more drug discontinuation in the placebo arm.

Although there are clear and compelling benefits with in-hospital initiation of SGLT2i, there is no consensus at which point during a hospitalization to initiate SGLT2i relative to other GDMT. Although some would point to the augmented diuresis with SGLT2i seen in the EMPA-RESPONSE-AHF trial as a reason to initiate as early as possible (before ARNi, BB, and MRA), this did not result in a shorter length of stay.[19] In EMPULSE, the median time of initiation was 3 days into admission with patients having to demonstrate clinical stability as evidenced by an SBP greater than 100 mm Hg, no symptomatic hypotension, no increase in intravenous (IV) diuretics or use of IV vasodilators within 6 h, and no IV ionotropic support within 24 h. Factors such as upcoming procedures, renal function, and adjustment of diabetes medications may also influence the timing of initiation.[41] Fortunately, as complete benefits of SGLT2i are obtained at the initial dosage, the main priority should simply be the initiation of the medication beforedischarge.

Initiation of GDMT in-hospital is crucially important with one in four patients dying or rehospitalized within 30 days of discharge of an HF hospitilizaiton.[42] In-hospital initiation of SGLT2i is safe and results in rapid clinical benefits that reduce hospitalization and death in the high-risk post-discharge period.

COST AND VALUE CONSIDERATIONS

SGLT2i are relatively new drugs on the market and as such will likely be under patent in the United States until at least 2025. Consequentially, out-of-pocket drug costs for SGLT2i, which can be upwards of $300 per month, are unaffordable for many patients without extra efforts to increase the accessiblity.[41] Because of additional time and resources needed to obtain SGLT2i for patients, clinicians may feel reluctant to use SGLT2i alongside other pillars of GDMT. Due to costs, hospitals and payers may avoid adding SGLT2i to covered formularies. However, these barriers are worth overcoming to realize the impressive morbidity and mortality benefit of the medication class. A cost-effectiveness analysis by Isaza and colleagues showed that in the United States, dapagliflozin costs $68,300 per quality-adjusted life year (QALY) gained.[43] This figure is far below the $150,000 per QALY threshold that the ACC/AHA set for low-value interventions and on par with ARNi, which also remain under patent.[44,45] Moreover, more frequent in-hospital initiation may further increase value due to a larger absolute risk reduction in the high-risk postdischarge period.[46] In the treatment of HF, where few medications have demonstrated mortality benefit and the four pillars of therapy have additive clinical benefit, it is the best interests of patients and the health care system to ensure access to SGLT2i.

SGLT2i USE IN PATIENTS WITH HEART FAILURE AND EJECTION FRACTION GREATER THAN 40%

Patients with HFmrEF and HFpEF have traditionally been a difficult patient population to treat.[47] RAASi, ARNi, and MRA may have modest benefits. However, SGLT2i have recently been shown in multiple trials to improve morbidity and symptoms across the entire EF spectrum of HF to a much greater degree than RAASi, ARNi, and MRA.[5,27,40]

The SOLOIST-WHF trial was the first to suggest the benefit of the SGLT inhibitor mechanism in patients with HFpEF.[40] In prespecified subgroup analysis of patients with EF $\geq$ 50%, sotagliflozin reduced the primary endpoint of cardiovascular death or urgent visits/hospitalizations for HF by

52% compared with placebo. Subsequently, the EMPEROR-Preserved trial, showed a 21% decrease in the primary outcome of cardiovascular death or HF hospitalization with empagliflozin versus placebo in patients with HF and an EF $\geq$ 40%.[5,48] This benefit reached statistical significance only 18 days after randomization. Of note, the reduction in the primary outcome was driven almost entirely from a reduction in HF hospitalizations. Additionally, in prespecified subgroup analysis, benefit was found across all EF ranges but was greatest in the EF $\leq$50% group. Unfortunately, both trials failed to achieve the elusive goal of all-cause mortality benefit with drug therapy in an HF population with EF greater than 40%. Even still, SGLT2i are an effective treatment to reduce HF hospitalizations for patients with HFmrEF or HFpEF. In the EMPULSE trial, the clinical benefits achieved were similar for patients with EF $\leq$40% and greater than 40% further demonstrating the benefits of SGLT2i therapy apply irrespective of EF group.[27] The totality of evidence suggests that early in-hospital initiation of SGLT2i should be the standard of care for patients with HF, irrespective of EF.

SUMMARY

SGLT2i are the newest member of the core HFrEF therapies that improve morbidity and mortality and accrue benefit within 30 days of initiation in large-scale RCTs. Initiation of SGLT2i should occur as soon as possible either in simultaneous or in rapid sequence with other GDMT agents. Furthermore, consideration for device therapy such as ICD, CRT, and TEER should wait until the initiation of SGLT2i. In-hospital initiation of SGLT2i is well tolerated and crucial given the risks of death and re-hospitalization after discharge and pervasive clinical inertia in the outpatient setting. SGLT2i are high-value medications, and efforts should be made to reduce acquisition costs for patients. More recent data favor initiation of SGLT2i in patients with HFmrEF/HFpEF to reduce the risk of hospitalization due to HF and demonstrates the benefits of early in-hospital initiation, irrespective of EF in patients hospitalized with HF.

CLINICS CARE POINTS

- SGLT2i demonstrate morbidity and mortality benefits within 30 days of initiation, possibly related to rapid reverse cardiac remodeling, reduced congestion, and increases in the cardioprotective and hematocrit-stimulating hormone, erythropoietin
- To maximize total relative risk reduction in morbidity and mortality, SGLT2i should be initiated simultaneously or in rapid sequence with the other core pillars of GDMT
- Due to LVEF and cardiac structure improvements induced by SGLT2i, consideration for device therapies such as ICD, CRT, and TEER should occur after SGLT2i initiation
- In-hospital initiation of SGLT2i is well tolerated and safe and reduces the risk of rehospitalization and death
- SGLT2i are lifesaving, high-value medications, and patient affordability is a key issue
- SGLT2i have more recently shown to reduce heart failure (HF) hospitalization in HF patients with EF greater than 40% and are a valuable potential therapy in a population with few therapeutic options

FUNDING

G.C. Fonarow recieves funding from the Ahmanson and Corday Foundations.

DISCLOSURE

Dr G.C. Fonarow has consulted for Abbott, Amgen, AstraZeneca, Bayer, Cytokinetics, Janssen, Medtronic, Merck, and Novartis. The rest of the authors declare no relevant conflicts of interest.

REFERENCES

1. Groenewegen A, Rutten FH, Mosterd A, et al. Epidemiology of heart failure. Eur J Heart Fail 2020;22(8): 1342–56.
2. Shah KS, Xu H, Matsouaka RA, et al. Heart Failure With Preserved, Borderline, and Reduced Ejection Fraction: 5-Year Outcomes. J Am Coll Cardiol 2017;70(20):2476–86.
3. Greene SJ, Butler J, Albert NM, et al. Medical Therapy for Heart Failure With Reduced Ejection Fraction: The CHAMP-HF Registry. J Am Coll Cardiol 2018;72(4):351–66.
4. Maddox TM, Januzzi JL, Allen LA, et al. 2021 Update to the 2017 ACC Expert Consensus Decision Pathway for Optimization of Heart Failure Treatment: Answers to 10 Pivotal Issues About Heart Failure With Reduced Ejection Fraction. J Am Coll Cardiol 2021;77(6):772–810.

5. Packer M, Butler J, Zannad F, et al. Effect of Empagliflozin on Worsening Heart Failure Events in Patients With Heart Failure and Preserved Ejection Fraction: EMPEROR-Preserved Trial. Circulation 2021;144(16):1284–94.

6. Monica Reddy RP, Inzucchi SE. SGLT2 inhibitors in the management of type 2 diabetes. Endocrine 2016;53(2):364–72.

7. Heerspink HJL, Stefánsson BV, Correa-Rotter R, et al. Dapagliflozin in Patients with Chronic Kidney Disease. N Engl J Med 2020;383(15):1436–46.

8. Zannad F, Ferreira JP, Pocock SJ, et al. SGLT2 inhibitors in patients with heart failure with reduced ejection fraction: a meta-analysis of the EMPEROR-Reduced and DAPA-HF trials. Lancet 2020; 396(10254):819–29.

9. Packer M, Anker SD, Butler J, et al. Effect of Empagliflozin on the Clinical Stability of Patients with Heart Failure and a Reduced Ejection Fraction: The EMPEROR-Reduced Trial. Circulation 2021. https://doi.org/10.1161/CIRCULATIONAHA.120.051783.

10. McMurray JJV, Solomon SD, Inzucchi SE, et al. Dapagliflozin in Patients with Heart Failure and Reduced Ejection Fraction. N Engl J Med 2019; 381(21):1995–2008.

11. Dixit N, Shah S, Ziaeian B, et al. Optimizing Guideline-directed Medical Therapies for Heart Failure with Reduced Ejection Fraction During Hospitalization. US Cardiology Review 2021;15:e07.

12. Berg DD, Jhund PS, Docherty KF, et al. Time to Clinical Benefit of Dapagliflozin and Significance of Prior Heart Failure Hospitalization in Patients With Heart Failure With Reduced Ejection Fraction. JAMA Cardiol 2021. https://doi.org/10.1001/jamacardio.2020.7585.

13. Lopaschuk GD, Verma S. Mechanisms of Cardiovascular Benefits of Sodium Glucose Co-Transporter 2 (SGLT2) Inhibitors: A State-of-the-Art Review. JACC Basic Transl Sci 2020;5(6):632–44.

14. Packer M. What causes sudden death in patients with chronic heart failure and a reduced ejection fraction? Eur Heart J 2019;41(18):1757–63.

15. Yancy CW, Jessup M, Bozkurt B, et al. 2013 ACCF/AHA guideline for the management of heart failure: a report of the American College of Cardiology Foundation/American Heart Association Task Force on Practice Guidelines. J Am Coll Cardiol 2013; 62(16):e147–239.

16. Santos-Gallego CG, Vargas-Delgado AP, Requena JA, et al. Randomized Trial of Empagliflozin in Non-Diabetic Patients with Heart Failure and Reduced Ejection Fraction. J Am Coll Cardiol 2020. https://doi.org/10.1016/j.jacc.2020.11.008.

17. Santos-Gallego Carlos G, Requena-Ibanez Juan A, San Antonio R, et al. Empagliflozin Ameliorates Adverse Left Ventricular Remodeling in Nondiabetic

Heart Failure by Enhancing Myocardial Energetics. J Am Coll Cardiol 2019;73(15):1931–44.

18. Burnier M, Brunner HR. Neurohormonal consequences of diuretics in different cardiovascular syndromes. Eur Heart J 1992;13(Suppl G):28–33.

19. Damman K, Beusekamp JC, Boorsma EM, et al. Randomized, double-blind, placebo-controlled, multicentre pilot study on the effects of empagliflozin on clinical outcomes in patients with acute decompensated heart failure (EMPA-RESPONSE-AHF). Eur J Heart Fail 2020;22(4):713–22.

20. Griffin M, Rao VS, Ivey-Miranda J, et al. Empagliflozin in Heart Failure. Circulation 2020;142(11): 1028–39.

21. Hartupee J, Mann DL. Neurohormonal activation in heart failure with reduced ejection fraction. Nat Rev Cardiol 2017;14(1):30–8.

22. Mazer CD, Hare GMT, Connelly PW, et al. Effect of Empagliflozin on Erythropoietin Levels, Iron Stores, and Red Blood Cell Morphology in Patients With Type 2 Diabetes Mellitus and Coronary Artery Disease. Circulation 2020;141(8):704–7.

23. Santhanam AV, d'Uscio LV, Katusic ZS. Cardiovascular effects of erythropoietin an update. Adv Pharmacol 2010;60:257–85.

24. Groenveld HF, Januzzi JL, Damman K, et al. Anemia and mortality in heart failure patients a systematic review and meta-analysis. J Am Coll Cardiol 2008; 52(10):818–27.

25. Greene SJ, Butler J, Fonarow GC. Simultaneous or Rapid Sequence Initiation of Quadruple Medical Therapy for Heart Failure-Optimizing Therapy With the Need for Speed. JAMA Cardiol 2021;6(7):743–4.

26. Docherty KF, Jhund PS, Inzucchi SE, et al. Effects of dapagliflozin in DAPA-HF according to background heart failure therapy. Eur Heart J 2020;41(25): 2379–92.

27. Voors AA, Angerman CE, Teerlink JR, et al. The SGLT2 inhibitor empagliflozin in patients hospitalized for acute heart failure: a multinational randomzied trial. Nat Med 2022;28(3):568–74.

28. Shen L, Kristensen SL, Bengtsson O, et al. Dapagliflozin in HFrEF Patients Treated With Mineralocorticoid Receptor Antagonists: An Analysis of DAPA-HF. JACC: Heart Fail 2021;9(4):254–64.

29. Ferreira JP, Zannad F, Pocock SJ, et al. Interplay of Mineralocorticoid Receptor Antagonists and Empagliflozin in Heart Failure: EMPEROR-Reduced. J Am Coll Cardiol 2021;77(11):1397–407.

30. Wheeler DC, Stefansson BV, Batiushin M, et al. The dapagliflozin and prevention of adverse outcomes in chronic kidney disease (DAPA-CKD) trial: baseline characteristics. Nephrol Dial Transpl 2020; 35(10):1700–11.

31. McGuire DK, Shih WJ, Cosentino F, et al. Association of SGLT2 Inhibitors With Cardiovascular and Kidney

Outcomes in Patients With Type 2 Diabetes: A Meta-analysis. JAMA Cardiol 2021;6(2):148–58.

32. Kario K, Ferdinand KC, Vongpatanasin W. Are SGLT2 Inhibitors New Hypertension Drugs? Circulation 2021;143(18):1750–3.

33. Böhm M, Anker Stefan D, Butler J, et al. Empagliflozin Improves Cardiovascular and Renal Outcomes in Heart Failure Irrespective of Systolic Blood Pressure. J Am Coll Cardiol 2021;78(13):1337–48.

34. Serenelli M, Böhm M, Inzucchi SE, et al. Effect of dapagliflozin according to baseline systolic blood pressure in the Dapagliflozin and Prevention of Adverse Outcomes in Heart Failure trial (DAPA-HF). Eur Heart J 2020;41(36):3402–18.

35. Rao VN, Murray E, Butler J, et al. In-Hospital Initiation of Sodium-Glucose Cotransporter-2 Inhibitors for Heart Failure With Reduced Ejection Fraction. J Am Coll Cardiol 2021;78(20):2004–12.

36. Otto CM, Nishimura RA, Bonow RO, et al. 2020 ACC/AHA Guideline for the Management of Patients With Valvular Heart Disease. J Am Coll Cardiol 2021. https://doi.org/10.1016/j.jacc.2020.11.018.

37. Bergethon KE, Ju C, DeVore AD, et al. Trends in 30-Day Readmission Rates for Patients Hospitalized With Heart Failure: Findings From the Get With The Guidelines-Heart Failure Registry. Circ Heart Fail 2016;9(6). https://doi.org/10.1161/circheartfailure.115.002594.

38. Pandey A, Patel KV, Liang L, et al. Association of Hospital Performance Based on 30-Day Risk-Standardized Mortality Rate With Long-term Survival After Heart Failure Hospitalization: An Analysis of the Get With The Guidelines-Heart Failure Registry. JAMA Cardiol 2018;3(6):489–97.

39. Packer M, Anker SD, Butler J, et al. Cardiovascular and Renal Outcomes with Empagliflozin in Heart Failure. N Engl J Med 2020;383(15):1413–24.

40. Bhatt DL, Szarek M, Steg PG, et al. Sotagliflozin in Patients with Diabetes and Recent Worsening Heart Failure. N Engl J Med 2021;384(2):117–28.

41. Honigberg MC, Vardeny O, Vaduganathan M. Practical Considerations for the Use of Sodium-Glucose Co-Transporter 2 Inhibitors in Heart Failure. Circ Heart Fail 2020;13(2):e006623.

42. Wadhera RK, Joynt Maddox KE, Wasfy JH, et al. Association of the Hospital Readmissions Reduction Program With Mortality Among Medicare Beneficiaries Hospitalized for Heart Failure, Acute Myocardial Infarction, and Pneumonia. Jama 2018;320(24):2542–52.

43. Isaza N, Calvachi P, Raber I, et al. Cost-effectiveness of Dapagliflozin for the Treatment of Heart Failure With Reduced Ejection Fraction. JAMA Netw Open 2021;4(7):e2114501.

44. Anderson JL, Heidenreich PA, Barnett PG, et al. ACC/AHA statement on cost/value methodology in clinical practice guidelines and performance measures: a report of the American College of Cardiology/American Heart Association Task Force on Performance Measures and Task Force on Practice Guidelines. J Am Coll Cardiol 2014;63(21):2304–22.

45. Gaziano TA, Fonarow GC, Claggett B, et al. Cost-effectiveness Analysis of Sacubitril/Valsartan vs Enalapril in Patients With Heart Failure and Reduced Ejection Fraction. JAMA Cardiol 2016;1(6):666–72.

46. Gaziano TA, Fonarow GC, Velazquez EJ, et al. Cost-effectiveness of Sacubitril-Valsartan in Hospitalized Patients Who Have Heart Failure With Reduced Ejection Fraction. JAMA Cardiol 2020. https://doi.org/10.1001/jamacardio.2020.2822.

47. Hsu JJ, Ziaeian B, Fonarow GC. Heart Failure With Mid-Range (Borderline) Ejection Fraction: Clinical Implications and Future Directions. JACC Heart Fail 2017;5(11):763–71.

48. Anker SD, Butler J, Filippatos G, et al. Empagliflozin in Heart Failure with a Preserved Ejection Fraction. N Engl J Med 2021;385(16):1451–61.

Sodium-Glucose Cotransporter-2 Inhibitors: Impact on Atherosclerosis and Atherosclerotic Cardiovascular Disease Events

Adam J. Nelson, MBBS, MBA, MPH, PhD[a], Josephine L. Harrington, MD[a],
Ahmed A. Kolkailah, MD, MSc[b], Neha J. Pagidipati, MD, MPH[a],
Darren K. McGuire, MD, MHSc[b,c],*

KEYWORDS

- Sodium-glucose cotransporter-2 inhibitors • Type 2 diabetes mellitus • Atherosclerosis
- Myocardial infarction • Stroke

KEY POINTS

- Sodium-glucose cotransporter-2 inhibitors (SGLT-2i) reduce the incidence of myocardial infarction by ~ 11% but do not seem to have an effect on stroke.
- Translational data suggest SGLT-2i may favorably affect plaque burden and composition through attenuation of inflammatory and cell adhesion pathways. However, human data are lacking.
- The individual postmarketing cardiovascular outcomes trials studied only patients with type 2 diabetes, so it is unclear if their results apply to patients without diabetes. In addition, all such trials were primarily designed to assess noninferiority (ie, safety) and were not specifically powered to determine the effectiveness of SGLT-2i on atherosclerotic events; further large studies are required.

INTRODUCTION

Sodium-glucose cotransporter-2 inhibitors (SGLT-2i) were initially developed as antihyperglycemic medications for the treatment of patients with type 2 diabetes mellitus (T2DM).[1] However, based on results from a series of postmarketing cardiovascular (CV) outcomes trials, their indications have expanded beyond simply lowering blood glucose. For those with T2DM with or at high risk for atherosclerotic cardiovascular disease (ASCVD), SGLT2i are now indicated for the prevention of multiple CV and kidney-related outcomes. Furthermore, SGLT2i are now indicated for patients with heart failure (HF) and/or chronic kidney disease (CKD), regardless of diabetes status.[2,3] Accordingly, SGLT-2i are now firmly established as medications capable of modifying the natural history of both HF and CKD, yet there is a paucity of synthesized evidence with regard to their impact on ASCVD events.[4] The aim of this review is to summarize the translational and clinical data evaluating the effects of SGLT-2i on ASCVD events with a particular focus on myocardial infarction (MI) and stroke.

[a] Duke Clinical Research Institute, 300 W Morgan Street, Durham, NC 27701, USA; [b] Division of Cardiology, University of Texas Southwestern Medical Center, Dallas, TX 75235-8830, USA; [c] Parkland Health and Hospital System, Dallas, TX, USA
* Corresponding author. Division of Cardiology, University of Texas Southwestern Medical Center, 5323 Harry Hines Boulevard, Dallas, TX 75235-8830.
E-mail address: darren.mcguire@utsouthwestern.edu

Heart Failure Clin 18 (2022) 597–607
https://doi.org/10.1016/j.hfc.2022.03.007
1551-7136/22/© 2022 Elsevier Inc. All rights reserved.

Evidence of Atherosclerotic Cardiovascular Disease Benefits of Sodium-Glucose Cotransporter-2 Inhibitor from Cardiovascular Clinical Outcomes Trials

Although limited to patients with T2DM, results from multiple, large, seminal CV outcomes trials provide the most robust clinical insights into the beneficial effects of SGLT-2i on major atherosclerotic cardiovascular disease (ASCVD) events.[4] These trials were randomized, double-blind, placebo-controlled parallel group studies with blinded and standardized event adjudication. Seven major outcomes trials have been performed with SGLT-2i in patients with T2DM (**Table 1**): The Empagliflozin Cardiovascular Outcome Event Trial in T2DM Patients–Removing Excess Glucose (EMPA-REG OUTCOME) evaluated empagliflozin versus placebo in 7020 patients for a median follow-up of 3.1 years[5]; the CANagliflozin cardioVascular Assessment Study (CANVAS) trials program comprised 2 trials (collectively known as the CANVAS trials program) and evaluated canagliflozin versus placebo in a total of 10,142 patients for a median follow-up of 2.4 years[6]; the Dapagliflozin Effect on CardiovascuLAR Events (DECLARE-thrombolysis in myocardial infarction [TIMI] 58) trial evaluated dapagliflozin versus placebo in 17,160 patients for a median follow-up of 4.2 years[7]; the Canagliflozin and Renal Events in Diabetes with Established Nephropathy Clinical Evaluation (CREDENCE) trial evaluated canagliflozin versus placebo in 4401 patients with underlying kidney dysfunction for a median follow-up of 2.6 years[8]; the Evaluation of Ertugliflozin Efficacy and Safety Cardiovascular Outcomes Trial (VERTIS CV) trial evaluated ertugliflozin versus placebo in 8230 patients for a median follow-up of 3.0 years[9]; and the Effect of Sotagliflozin on Cardiovascular and Renal Events in Patients with Type 2 Diabetes and moderate Renal Impairment who are at Cardiovascular Risk (SCORED) trial evaluated sotagliflozin versus placebo in 10,584 patients for a median follow-up of 16 months after it was terminated prematurely due to loss of funding.[10] EMPA-REG OUTCOME, CANVAS, DECLARE-TIMI 58, and VERTIS CV all used a 3-point major atherosclerotic cardiovascular event (MACE) primary outcome comprising the time to first CV death, nonfatal MI, or nonfatal stroke, whereas CREDENCE included MACE as a prioritized secondary outcome (see **Table 1**). Although this MACE composite is generally considered an "atherosclerotic" outcome, the definition of CV death also includes death due to arrhythmia, HF, CV procedure complication, and CV hemorrhage and thus is not necessarily exclusively related to atherosclerosis.

Each of these trials exclusively enrolled patients with T2DM, enriched for patients with—or at high risk for—ASCVD. As a result, baseline prevalence of ASCVD in these trials ranged from 40% in DECLARE-TIMI 58% to 100% in EMPA-REG OUTCOME and VERTIS CV. Similarly, ~20% of patients enrolled in DECLARE-TIMI 58 and ~50% of those enrolled in EMPA-REG OUTCOME and VERTIS CV had a prior MI. Baseline prevalence of prior MI was not reported for the CANVAS trials program or for CREDENCE. Consistent with these patient characteristics, both EMPA-REG OUTCOME and VERTIS CV had higher baseline use of antiplatelet and low-density lipoprotein cholesterol (LDL-C) lowering therapies at around 80% for each, whereas in DECLARE-TIMI 58, this was ~60% for antiplatelet and ~75% for LDL-C lowering therapies.

Sodium-glucose cotransporter-2 inhibitor effects on time-to-first cardiovascular death, myocardial infarction, or stroke

Compared with placebo-treated patients, a statistically significant reduction in the time-to-first MACE (defined as CV death, MI, or stroke) was observed among empagliflozin-treated patients in EMPA-REG OUTCOME (HR 0.86, 95%CI 0.74–0.99), canagliflozin-treated patients in both the CANVAS program (HR 0.86, 95%CI 0.75–0.97) and CREDENCE trial (0.80, 95%CI 0.67–0.95), in addition to sotagliflozin-treated patients in SCORED (HR 0.84, 95%CI 0.72–0.99). Statistically significant reductions compared with placebo were neither observed among dapagliflozin-treated patients in DECLARE-TIMI 58 (HR 0.93, 95%CI 0.84–1.03) nor among ertugliflozin-treated patients in VERTIS CV (HR 0.99, 95%CI 0.88–1.12). Random effects meta-analysis of all 6 programs revealed an overall 12% reduction in MACE (HR 0.88, 95%CI 0.83–0.93) with some observed heterogeneity that did not reach statistical significance (I^2 21%, $P = 0.19$).[11] Explanations for the difference of results with regard to MACE effects across the class and across the trials remain unclear, and may relate to agent-specific differences or the play of chance.

Sodium-glucose cotransporter-2 inhibitor effects on myocardial infarction

Analyzing the secondary outcome of time-to-first nonfatal MI, there was no statistical difference for SGLT-2i versus placebo in any of the individual trial programs. Specifically, the following results were observed for nonfatal MI: empagliflozin versus placebo in EMPA-REG OUTCOME, HR 0.87 (95% CI 0.70–1.09); canagliflozin vs placebo in (a) the CANVAS trials program, HR 0.89 (95% CI 0.77–1.01), and (b) in CREDENCE, HR 0.86

Table 1
Summary of the large CV outcomes trials of SGLT-2i

	EMPA-REG OUTCOME[5]	CANVAS Trials Program[6]	DECLARE-TIMI 58[7]	CREDENCE[8]	VERTIS CV[9]	SCORED[10]
Compound	Empagliflozin	Canagliflozin	Dapagliflozin	Canagliflozin	Ertugliflozin	Sotagliflozin
Published, year	2015	2017	2019	2019	2020	2021
Sample size, N	7020	10,142	17,160	4401	8238	10,584
Median FU, years	3.1	2.4	4.2	2.6	3.0	1.3
T2DM, %	100	100	100	100	100	100
Established ASCVD, %	99.2	72.2	40.6	50.4	100	48.6
Prior MI, %	46.4	NR	20.9	NR	47.9	20.0
PAD, %	21.5	20.8	6	23.8	18.6	NR
Baseline LDL-C, mg/dL	85.9	88.9	NR	96.4	89.3	NR
CVD medications, %						
Antiplatelet	82.7	73.6	61.1	59.6	84.5	NR
Statin/ezetimibe	77.0	74.9	75.0	69.0	82.3	NR
Primary outcome	CV death, nonfatal MI, nonfatal stroke	CV death, nonfatal MI, nonfatal stroke	CV death, nonfatal MI, nonfatal stroke	ESKD, doubling of serum creatinine, kidney/CV death	CV death, nonfatal MI, nonfatal stroke	CV death, nonfatal MI, nonfatal stroke
MACE						
Events in trial	490 (10.5) vs 282 (12.1)	NA	756 (8.8) vs 803 (9.4)	217 (9.9) vs 269 (12.2)	735 (13.4) vs 368 (13.4)	286 (5.4) vs 334 (6.3)
Rate/1000 pt yrs	27.4 vs 43.9	26.9 vs 31.5	22.6 vs 24.2	38.7 vs 48.7	40.0 vs 40.3	40.5 vs 47.3
HR (95%CI)	0.86 (0.74–0.99)	0.86 (0.75–0.97)	0.93 (0.84–1.03)	0.80 (0.67–0.95)	0.99 (0.88–1.12)	0.84 (0.72–0.99)
CV death						
Events in trial	172 (3.7) vs 137 (5.9)	NA	245 (2.9) vs 249 (2.9)	110 (5.0) vs 140 (6.4)	341 (6.2) vs 184 (7.4)	155 (2.9) vs 170 (3.2)
Rate/1000 pt yrs	12.4 vs 20.2	11.6 vs 12.8	7.0 vs 7.1	19.0 vs 24.4	17.6 vs 19.0	22.0 vs 24.0
HR (95%CI)	0.62 (0.49–0.77)	0.87 (0.72–1.06)	0.98 (0.82–1.17)	0.78 (0.61–1.00)	0.92 (0.77–1.10)	0.90 (0.73–1.12)

(continued on next page)

Table 1
(continued)

	EMPA-REG OUTCOME[5]	CANVAS Trials Program[6]	DECLARE-TIMI 58[7]	CREDENCE[8]	VERTIS CV[9]	SCORED[10]
MI						
Events in trial	223 (4.5) vs 126 (5.2)	NA	393 (4.6) vs 441 (5.1)	83 (3.8) vs 95 (4.3)	330 (6.0) vs 158 (5.8)	NR
Rate/1000 pt yrs	16.8 vs 19.3	11.2 vs 12.6	11.7 vs 13.2	14.6 vs 16.9	17.7 vs 17.0	NR
HR (95%CI)	0.87 (0.70–1.09)	0.89 (0.73–1.09)	0.89 (0.77–1.01)	0.86 (0.64–1.16)	1.04 (0.86–1.26)	0.68 (0.52–0.89)[a]
Stroke						
Events in trial	164 (3.5) vs 69 (3.0)	NA	NA	62 (2.8) vs 80 (3.6)	185 (3.4%) vs 87 (3.2%)	NR
Rate/1000 pt yrs	12.3 vs 10.5	7.9 vs 9.6	7.5 vs 7.8	10.9 vs 14.2	9.8 vs 9.3	NR
HR 95%CI	1.18 (0.89–1.56)	0.87 (0.69–1.09)	0.96 (0.81–1.14)	0.77 (0.55–1.08)	1.06 (0.87–1.07)	0.66 (0.48–0.91)[a]
Amputations						
Events in trial	88 (1.9) vs 43 (1.8)	140 (2.4) vs 47 (1.1)	123 (1.4) vs 113 (1.3)	70 (3.2) vs 63 (2.9)	101 (1.8) vs 45 (1.6)	NR
Rate/1000 pt yrs	6.1 vs 5.9	NA	3.4 vs 3.2	12.2 vs 11.0	6.1 vs 5.5	NR
HR 95%CI	1.02 (0.71–1.46)	2.23 (1.61–3.10)	1.09 (0.84–1.40)	1.11 (0.79–1.55)	1.12 (0.79–1.59)	NR

Abbreviations: ASCVD, atherosclerotic cardiovascular disease; CV, cardiovascular; ESKD, end-stage kidney disease; FU, follow up; LDL-C, low-density lipoprotein cholesterol; MACE, major adverse cardiovascular events; MI, myocardial infarction; NR, not recorded; PAD, peripheral artery disease; pt yrs, patient-years; T2DM, type 2 diabetes mellitus.
[a] Total events rather than first events.

(95% CI 0.64–1.16); dapagliflozin versus placebo in DECLARE-TIMI 58, HR 0.89 (95% CI 0.73–1.09); and ertugliflozin versus placebo in VERTIS CV, HR 1.04 (95% CI 0.86–1.26). However, in an exploratory, post hoc analysis that was not adjusted for multiplicity, and therefore must be interpreted with caution, sotagliflozin-treated patients experienced fewer total fatal and nonfatal MIs; HR 0.68 (95% CI 0.52–0.89). Meta-analysis of all 6 programs that included the total events analysis from SCORED, yielded an overall 11% nominally significant, relative reduction in the hazard of nonfatal MI compared with placebo (HR 0.89, 95% CI 0.82–0.96).[11]

A network meta-analysis of randomized controlled trials performed until October 2017, Zheng and colleagues included studies of at least 12 weeks duration that compared SGLT-2i, glucagon-like receptor agonists and dipeptidyl-peptidase 4 inhibitors (DPP-4i) with each other or placebo or no treatment.[12] The overall study included 236 trials randomizing 176,310 participants. However, for the outcome of all MIs, 19,958 SGLT-2i-treated patients from 32 trials were included with overall low heterogeneity (I^2 = 15%). SGLT-2i-treated patients had a 14% lower relative risk for all MIs compared with control (HR 0.86, 95%CI 0.77–0.97) equating to an absolute risk difference of −0.6% between arms. Given the neutrality of DPP-4i with respect to MI, comparison between SGLT-2i and DPP-4i is of interest as a form of active comparator control. Comparing these 2 agents in the network meta-analysis, there was evidence of a similar magnitude of benefit favoring SGLT-2i, although this did not reach statistical significance (HR 0.91, 95%CI 0.80–1.04).

In the context of clinical trials powered for ASCVD safety but not necessarily efficacy assessments, observational data can provide valuable insights into the effects of SGLT-2i in clinical practice. In this context, the Comparative Effectiveness of Cardiovascular Outcomes in New Users of SGLT-2 Inhibitors (CVD REAL) registry is a multinational aggregated dataset of deidentified health records from 13 countries.[13] Participants with T2DM were identified through internationational classification of diseases (ICD) codes and were considered eligible for this study if commencing either an SGLT-2i or DPP-4i during 2012 through 2016. Propensity score matching was performed to balance baseline characteristics with MACE outcomes collected through medical record encounters. Mean age of the cohort was 57 years with approximately 30% reporting an ASCVD history. In the propensity-matched cohort of 386,248 participants (193,124 in each group), new commencers of SGLT-2i (dapagliflozin was

the SGLT-2i in 60% of the cohort) had a significantly lower risk of incident MI compared with those commencing DPP-4i (HR 0.88, 95%CI 0.80–0.98). The strengths of this analysis are its multinational experience, longer duration of follow-up (421,232 person years), new-user design, and enrollment of an overall lower-risk group than the regulatory trials (event rate ∼ 5/1000 person years). The weaknesses include the potential for residual confounding and incomplete, unadjudicated event ascertainment.

Sodium-glucose cotransporter-2 inhibitor effects on nonfatal stroke

There seems to be minimal, if any, consistent effect of SGLT-2i on the incidence of stroke. Numerically fewer stroke events were observed in patients randomized to canagliflozin in both the CREDENCE (10.9 vs 14.2 events/1000 patient years; HR 0.77, 95%CI 0.55–1.08) and CANVAS programs (7.9 vs 9.6 events/1000 patient years; HR 0.87, 95%CI 0.69–1.09). However, neither reached statistical significance and these signals were not observed in EMPA-REG OUTCOME (HR 1.18, 95% CI 0.89–1.56), DECLARE-TIMI 58 (HR 0.98, 95%CI 0.82–1.17) or VERTIS CV (HR 1.06, 95% CI 0.87–1.07). In exploratory, post hoc analyses from SCORED, not adjusted for multiplicity, sotagliflozin-treated patients experienced fewer total (rather than time-to-first-event) strokes compared with placebo (HR 0.66, 95%CI 0.48–0.91). Even with SCORED included in the pooled results, the overall meta-analysis did not show a significant treatment effect of SGLT2i on stroke (HR 0.92, 95% CI 0.79–1.08).[11] Of note, in the CV outcome trials of SGLT-2i in patients with T2DM and ASCVD or high ASCVD risk, ischemic and hemorrhagic events were included in the key stroke outcome as defined in the adjudication charter of each trial, making it impracticable to parse out the presence or absence of an SGLT-2i effect on ischemic stroke. This nonspecific definition of stroke by cause, in addition to the fact stroke is a less common event than ischemic heart disease events, and thus more sensitive to noise, may underpin the heterogeneity of observed results from the outcome trials.

In the Zheng meta-analysis, which included 15,333 patients from 30 trials, the 243 stroke events (1.6%) were nearly balanced across the SGLT-2i and control arms (HR 0.92, 95%CI 0.79–1.08). In contrast, the results from observational data diverge and are more supportive of a salutary effect on stroke. In the CVD REAL observational registry, there were 3821 stroke events (overall rate of 10 per 1000 patient years), which were less common among SGLT-2i commencing patients compared with those commencing DPP-4i

(HR 0.85, 95%CI 0.77–0.93). No significant interaction was noted among those with CVD at baseline compared with those without CVD at baseline (P = 0.30). Of note, before propensity matching, the patients commencing SGLT-2i were younger with lower rates of AF and prior stroke, so unmeasured residual confounding may be contributing to the observed effects.

Sodium-glucose co-transporter-2 inhibitor effects on unstable angina and coronary revascularization

Rates of other atherosclerotic outcomes like revascularization and unstable angina have not been consistently reported in the larger trials and were not subject to blinded adjudication. In the Zheng meta-analysis that included 16 trials that reported unstable angina, there were 154 events with no obvious effect of SGLT-2i compared with controls (HR 0.91, 95%CI 0.74–1.27).[12] These results need to be interpreted with caution as the definitions for the events varied considerably among the included studies and the attribution of an event-like unstable angina in the absence of blinded and standardized adjudication is inherently subjective. However, these events affect the quality of life and are patient-centered and thus ought to be considered in future studies aimed to evaluate the totality of SGLT-2i effects on atherosclerotic events.

Sodium-glucose cotransporter-2 inhibitor effects on atherosclerotic events in the absence of type 2 diabetes mellitus

Although several trials have deliberately enrolled patients without T2DM in order to determine the effect of SGLT-2i on kidney[14] and HF[15–17] outcomes, none of these studies were powered to determine their impact on atherosclerotic outcomes. Specifically, none of the HF trials (Dapagliflozin and Prevention of Adverse Outcomes in Heart Failure [DAPA HF], Empagliflozin Outcome Trial in Patients with Chronic Heart Failure with Reduced Ejection Fraction [EMPEROR-Reduced], and Empagliflozin Outcome Trial in Patients with Chronic Heart Failure with Preserved Ejection Fraction [EMPEROR-Preserved]) included MACE as an outcome in the primary hierarchy of analyses. The Dapagliflozin and Prevention of Adverse Outcomes in CKD (DAPA CKD) trial included a 3-point MACE (CV death, MI, and stroke) as a prespecified, exploratory outcome. However, the incidence of and comparative efficacy of dapagliflozin for this outcome have not been presented by T2DM status, and given that MACE occurred in only 3% of the trial cohort, there

is likely to be insufficient power for meaningful MACE analyses stratified by T2DM status.[18]

Translational Evidence Behind Potential Mechanisms of Benefit

Lipids

Data on the effect of SGLT-2i on the lipid profile are conflicting.[19] A meta-analysis of 48 RCTs comprising 22,156 participants reported an overall small increase in total cholesterol (weighted mean difference [WMD] +0.09 mmol/L), high-density lipoprotein-cholesterol (HDL-C) (WMD +0.06 mol/L) and LDL-C levels (WMD +0.1 mmol/L), and a small reduction in triglyceride levels (WMD −0.1 mmol/L).[20] Although these comparisons were statistically significant, there was considerable heterogeneity in the direction of these effects (I^2 all >90%), and the magnitude of these changes were too small to be of clinical importance.

Inflammation

Results from basic and in vivo studies suggest SGLT-2i may ameliorate several proinflammatory pathways related to atherosclerosis, with generally consistent effects in both patients with and without diabetes. Cellular data have shown SGLT-2i administration attenuates secretion of proinflammatory cytokines associated with early atherosclerosis including interleukin (IL)-6 and monocyte chemoattractant protein-1 cytokines, and upstream IL-1β,[21–23] and promote an anti-inflammatory macrophage phenotype.[23,24] In murine models of atherosclerosis and type 1 diabetes, SGLT-2i administration has been shown to reduce the expression of a variety of inflammation-related genes or their proteins (F4/80, IL-1β, tumor necrosis factor-alpha, IL-6, intracellular adhesion molecule (ICAM)-1, platelet endothelial cell adhesion molecule-1 (PECAM-1), matrix metalloproteinase (MMP2), MMP9) in aortic tissue,[25] plaques,[26–28] and perivascular adipose tissue.[26] Other animal and human studies have shown reductions in inflammatory activity of SGLT-2i treated animals with reduced subsequent activation of the innate inflammatory cascade.[27,29,30]

Vascular/endothelial cell function and oxidative stress

Multiple levels of evidence suggest that SGLT-2 inhibition results in salutary effects on endothelial dysfunction, oxidative stress, and leukocyte migration. Basic and animal models have shown SGLT-2i administration can reduce levels of reactive oxygen species (ROS), increase nitric oxide formation, and reverse diabetes-induced endothelial senescence.[31–33] Plaque of SGLT-2i-treated animals exhibits reduced expression of nicotin-amide adenine dinucleotide phosphate (NADPH) oxidases with attendant reduction in the levels of intermediate markers of oxidative stress (superoxide dismutase 2 (SOD2), thioredoxin (TXN), heme oxygenase 1 (HO1), leukocyte-dependent oxidative burst) in the presence and absence of hyperglycemia.[28,34,35] Atherosclerosis-prone mice treated with SGLT-2i exhibit reduced expression of vascular cell adhesion molecule-1 and ICAM-1, both of which are associated with early phases of inflammation, endothelial dysfunction and atherogenesis.[25,36] In vitro studies have also shown reduced (proinflammatory) IL-17A induced smooth muscle cell proliferation and migration.[37]

The direct effect of SGLT-2i on vascular function is less clear. Although results from animal studies suggest some potential improvement in microcirculatory function,[38,39] human studies evaluating changes in flow-mediated dilatation and markers of arterial stiffness such as pulse wave velocity have been conflicting[40–44] and may instead relate to associated changes in blood pressure or body weight.[45–49]

Plaque burden and characteristics
Animal models have shown SGLT-2i can reduce atherosclerotic plaque number and size,[50] with conflicting data as to the role of diabetes in these observations.[21,25,51,52] Whether SGLT-2i modifies the propensity for plaque formation to a greater degree in the presence of glycemia/diabetes status, or whether this relates to the length of SGLT-2i treatment remains unclear. Beyond plaque size, there is emerging evidence that SGLT-2i use generates plaque stability by modifying plaque characteristics and composition. Animal models have shown reduced plaque macrophage infiltration, fewer cholesterol crystals, and a switch

in the balance of matrix metalloproteinase activity to a less active, procollagenous and inert phenotype in the setting of SGLT-2i administration.[27,36,51,53] In a propensity-matched analysis of patients undergoing endarterectomy, plaque removed from patients treated with an SGLT-2i (n = 87) had higher expression of the anti-inflammatory SIRT6 and greater collagen content compared with patients not on an SGLT-2i (n = 87).[54]

Myocardial oxygen supply/demand
SGLT-2i modulate several cardiac parameters and pathways known to impact myocardial oxygen supply and demand, which in the context of ASCVD, may increase ischemic thresholds and reduce infarct size. A reduction in intravascular volume observed with SGLT-2i administration modestly reduces blood pressure without increasing the heart rate, likely confers reduced preload and cardiac work and, conceivably, reduces myocardial oxygen demand.[55] A blunting of the sympathetic nervous system likely underlies some of these benefits and may relate to ketosis-induced changes in vagal nerve activity,[56] favorable neurohormonal modulation induced by kidney recovery,[57] or direct action at the adrenal gland which seems to express SGLT-2i and may subsequently inhibit catecholamine biosynthesis[58] (Fig. 1).

Future directions
Almost all of the supportive translational data evaluating the impact of SGLT-2i is in atheroma-prone mouse or rat models. Although these models have been transformational in aiding our pathologic understanding of atherosclerosis, they are necessarily short-term and accelerated (occurring over weeks and months), and therefore do not

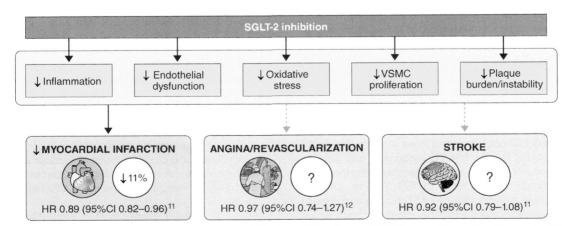

Fig. 1. Translational evidence supporting potentially favorable effects of SGLT2-i on atherosclerotic events. HR, hazard ratio; VSMC, vascular smooth muscle cell.

adequately recapitulate the acute (plaque event) on chronic pathophysiology seen in humans. Further, most murine studies induce diabetes through a mechanism that more closely mimics type 1 diabetes (that of insulin absence) and thus may not fully reflect the more common form of T2DM (that of insulin resistance). The current human clinical data in aggregate support the potential beneficial effects of SGLT-2i on MI. However, none of the individual trials definitively demonstrated this benefit. Most atherosclerotic events accrue beyond 18 months; thus, trials targeting an atherosclerotic outcome tend to have a median follow-up of at least 3.5 years to generate sufficient events and power to demonstrate superiority (eg, Canakinumab Anti-inflammatory Thrombosis Outcome Study – 3.7 years,[59] Reduction of Cardiovascular Events with Icosapent Ethyl–Intervention Trial – 4.9 years,[60] Improved Reduction of Outcomes: Vytorin Efficacy International Trial – 6 years[61]). Because many outcomes trials for SGLT-2is were intended to assess for CV safety, they were conducted as noninferiority trials and likely too short to demonstrate benefit, if one exists.

Furthermore, there is a complete absence of randomized data on the atherosclerotic clinical outcomes of patients treated with SGLT-2i in the absence of T2DM. There is an opportunity (and need) to randomize patients with ASCVD without T2DM (with potentially some other enriching metabolic risk factors such as obesity or dyslipidemia) to SGLT-2i or placebo, and powering for an atherosclerotic superiority assessment. To have 80% power, a study of this nature would require enrollment of ~15,000 patients to detect a 15% reduction in MACE at a baseline event rate of ~8%. Ideally, an outcomes study of this size would be complemented with a vascular wall imaging substudy (either computed tomography and/or positron-emission tomography), which would allow an evaluation of changes in plaque burden/activity and facilitate bridging of the current translational research gaps.

SUMMARY

The aggregate clinical data suggest that SGLT-2i have a robust safety profile with regard to effects on ASCVD outcomes but have modest effects on improving risk for ASCVD outcomes, with heterogeneity of effects across the class. Further randomized clinical trials of SGLT-2i in patients with—or at high risk of—ASCVD are required to adequately understand the effect of these drugs on ASCVD events and better inform clinical decision-making.

CLINICS CARE POINTS

- Sodium-glucose cotransporter-2 inhibitor (SGLT-2i) reduce major atherosclerotic cardiovascular event in the presence and absence of established atherosclerotic cardiovascular disease, independent of metformin use and regardless of baseline or achieved HbA1c.

- SGLT-2i can be commenced safely during hospitalization for decompensated heart failure—ongoing studies will determine whether the same is definitively true for myocardial infarction. However, in-hospital commencement is likely to be safe and provides an important opportunity to achieve guideline-recommended care among high-risk patients.

- If fasting for an interventional cardiovascular procedure, the risk for euglycemic ketoacidosis can be reduced by holding the SGLT-2i on the day of procedure and recommencing when the patient has returned to normal oral intake.

DISCLOSURE

A.J. Nelson—nothing to disclose; Josephine Harrington—completed work for this article while grant (T32HL069749); A.A. Kolkailah—was supported by the National Heart, Lung, and Blood Institute of the National Institutes of Health under Award Number T32HL12547. The content is solely the responsibility of the authors and does not necessarily represent the official view of the National Institutes of Health; N.J. Pagidipati - Grants from Amgen, Novartis, Novo Nordisk, Boehringer Ingelheim, Eli Lilly & Co, Cleerly, Eggland's Best, and Verily Life Sciences; personal fees from Boehringer Ingelheim, Eli Lilly & Co, Novo Nordisk, Novartis; D.K. McGuire - Personal fees from Boehringer Ingelheim, Sanofi US, Merck., Merck Sharp and Dohme., Eli Lilly & Co USA, Novo Nordisk, AstraZeneca, Lexicon Pharmaceuticals, Eisai, Pfizer, Metavant, Applied Therapeutics, Afimmune, Bayer, CSL Behring and Esperion.

REFERENCES

1. Nelson AJ, Pagidipati NJ, Aroda VR, et al. Incorporating SGLT2i and GLP-1RA for cardiovascular and kidney disease risk reduction: call for action to the cardiology community. Circulation 2021;144(1):74–84.

2. Packer M, Butler J, Zannad F, et al. Empagliflozin and major renal outcomes in heart failure. N Engl J Med 2021;385(16):1531–3.

3. Heerspink HJL, Jongs N, Chertow GM, et al. Effect of dapagliflozin on the rate of decline in kidney function in patients with chronic kidney disease with and without type 2 diabetes: a prespecified analysis from the DAPA-CKD trial. Lancet Diabetes Endocrinol 2021;9(11):743–54.

4. McGuire DK, Shih WJ, Cosentino F, et al. Association of SGLT2 inhibitors with cardiovascular and kidney outcomes in patients with type 2 diabetes: a meta-analysis. JAMA Cardiol 2021;6(2):148–58.

5. Zinman B, Wanner C, Lachin JM, et al. Empagliflozin, cardiovascular outcomes, and mortality in type 2 diabetes. N Engl J Med 2015;373(22):2117–28.

6. Neal B, Perkovic V, Mahaffey KW, et al. Canagliflozin and cardiovascular and renal events in type 2 diabetes. N Engl J Med 2017;377(7):644–57.

7. Wiviott SD, Raz I, Bonaca MP, et al. Dapagliflozin and cardiovascular outcomes in type 2 diabetes. N Engl J Med 2019;380(4):347–57.

8. Perkovic V, Jardine MJ, Neal B, et al. Canagliflozin and renal outcomes in type 2 diabetes and nephropathy. N Engl J Med 2019;380(24):2295–306.

9. Cannon CP, Pratley R, Dagogo-Jack S, et al. Cardiovascular outcomes with ertugliflozin in type 2 diabetes. N Engl J Med 2020;383(15):1425–35.

10. Bhatt DL, Szarek M, Pitt B, et al. Sotagliflozin in patients with diabetes and chronic kidney disease. N Engl J Med 2021;384(2):129–39.

11. Salah HM, Al'Aref SJ, Khan MS, et al. Effects of sodium-glucose cotransporter 1 and 2 inhibitors on cardiovascular and kidney outcomes in type 2 diabetes: a meta-analysis update. Am Heart J 2021; 233:86–91.

12. Zheng SL, Roddick AJ, Aghar-Jaffar R, et al. Association between use of sodium-glucose cotransporter 2 inhibitors, glucagon-like peptide 1 agonists, and dipeptidyl peptidase 4 inhibitors with all-cause mortality in patients with type 2 diabetes: a systematic review and meta-analysis. JAMA 2018;319(15): 1580–91.

13. Kohsaka S, Lam CSP, Kim DJ, et al. Risk of cardiovascular events and death associated with initiation of SGLT2 inhibitors compared with DPP-4 inhibitors: an analysis from the CVD-REAL 2 multinational cohort study. Lancet Diabetes Endocrinol 2020; 8(7):606–15.

14. Heerspink HJL, Stefansson BV, Correa-Rotter R, et al. Dapagliflozin in patients with chronic kidney disease. N Engl J Med 2020;383(15):1436–46.

15. Anker SD, Butler J, Filippatos G, et al. Empagliflozin in heart failure with a preserved ejection fraction. N Engl J Med 2021;385(16):1451–61.

16. McMurray JJV, Solomon SD, Inzucchi SE, et al. Dapagliflozin in patients with heart failure and reduced ejection fraction. N Engl J Med 2019;381(21): 1995–2008.

17. Packer M, Anker SD, Butler J, et al. Cardiovascular and renal outcomes with empagliflozin in heart failure. N Engl J Med 2020;383(15):1413–24.

18. McMurray JJV, Wheeler DC, Stefansson BV, et al. Effect of dapagliflozin on clinical outcomes in patients with chronic kidney disease, with and without cardiovascular disease. Circulation 2021;143(5): 438–48.

19. Storgaard H, Gluud LL, Bennett C, et al. Benefits and harms of sodium-glucose co-transporter 2 inhibitors in patients with type 2 diabetes: a systematic review and meta-analysis. PLoS One 2016; 11(11):e0166125.

20. Sanchez-Garcia A, Simental-Mendia M, Millan-Alanis JM, et al. Effect of sodium-glucose co-transporter 2 inhibitors on lipid profile: a systematic review and meta-analysis of 48 randomized controlled trials. Pharmacol Res 2020;160:105068.

21. Han JH, Oh TJ, Lee G, et al. The beneficial effects of empagliflozin, an SGLT2 inhibitor, on atherosclerosis in ApoE (-/-) mice fed a western diet. Diabetologia 2017;60(2):364–76.

22. Mancini SJ, Boyd D, Katwan OJ, et al. Canagliflozin inhibits interleukin-1beta-stimulated cytokine and chemokine secretion in vascular endothelial cells by AMP-activated protein kinase-dependent and -independent mechanisms. Sci Rep 2018;8(1):5276.

23. Xu C, Wang W, Zhong J, et al. Canagliflozin exerts anti-inflammatory effects by inhibiting intracellular glucose metabolism and promoting autophagy in immune cells. Biochem Pharmacol 2018;152:45–59.

24. Hess DA, Terenzi DC, Trac JZ, et al. SGLT2 Inhibition with empagliflozin increases circulating provascular progenitor cells in people with type 2 diabetes mellitus. Cell Metab 2019;30(4):609–13.

25. Nakatsu Y, Kokubo H, Bumdelger B, et al. The SGLT2 inhibitor luseogliflozin rapidly normalizes aortic mrna levels of inflammation-related but not lipid-metabolism-related genes and suppresses atherosclerosis in diabetic ApoE KO mice. Int J Mol Sci 2017;18(8).

26. Ganbaatar B, Fukuda D, Shinohara M, et al. Empagliflozin ameliorates endothelial dysfunction and suppresses atherogenesis in diabetic apolipoprotein E-deficient mice. Eur J Pharmacol 2020;875: 173040.

27. Leng W, Ouyang X, Lei X, et al. The SGLT-2 inhibitor dapagliflozin has a therapeutic effect on atherosclerosis in diabetic ApoE(-/-) mice. Mediators Inflamm 2016;2016:6305735.

28. Rahadian A, Fukuda D, Salim HM, et al. Canagliflozin prevents diabetes-induced vascular dysfunction in apoe-deficient mice. J Atheroscler Thromb 2020; 27(11):1141–51.

29. Kim SR, Lee SG, Kim SH, et al. SGLT2 inhibition modulates NLRP3 inflammasome activity via

ketones and insulin in diabetes with cardiovascular disease. Nat Commun 2020;11(1):2127.

30. Ye Y, Bajaj M, Yang HC, et al. SGLT-2 inhibition with dapagliflozin reduces the activation of the Nlrp3/ASC inflammasome and attenuates the development of diabetic cardiomyopathy in mice with type 2 diabetes. further augmentation of the effects with saxagliptin, a DPP4 inhibitor. Cardiovasc Drugs Ther 2017;31(2):119–32.

31. Park SH, Belcastro E, Hasan H, et al. Angiotensin II-induced upregulation of SGLT1 and 2 contributes to human microparticle-stimulated endothelial senescence and dysfunction: protective effect of gliflozins. Cardiovasc Diabetol 2021;20(1):65.

32. Spigoni V, Fantuzzi F, Carubbi C, et al. Sodium-glucose cotransporter 2 inhibitors antagonize lipotoxicity in human myeloid angiogenic cells and ADP-dependent activation in human platelets: potential relevance to prevention of cardiovascular events. Cardiovasc Diabetol 2020;19(1):46.

33. Uthman L, Homayr A, Juni RP, et al. Empagliflozin and dapagliflozin reduce ROS Generation and restore no bioavailability in tumor necrosis factor alpha-stimulated human coronary arterial endothelial cells. Cell Physiol Biochem 2019;53(5):865–86.

34. Oelze M, Kroller-Schon S, Welschof P, et al. The sodium-glucose co-transporter 2 inhibitor empagliflozin improves diabetes-induced vascular dysfunction in the streptozotocin diabetes rat model by interfering with oxidative stress and glucotoxicity. PLoS One 2014;9(11):e112394.

35. Steven S, Oelze M, Hanf A, et al. The SGLT2 inhibitor empagliflozin improves the primary diabetic complications in ZDF rats. Redox Biol 2017;13:370–85.

36. Nasiri-Ansari N, Dimitriadis GK, Agrogiannis G, et al. Canagliflozin attenuates the progression of atherosclerosis and inflammation process in APOE knockout mice. Cardiovasc Diabetol 2018;17(1):106.

37. Sukhanov S, Higashi Y, Yoshida T, et al. The SGLT2 inhibitor Empagliflozin attenuates interleukin-17A-induced human aortic smooth muscle cell proliferation and migration by targeting TRAF3IP2/ROS/NLRP3/Caspase-1-dependent IL-1beta and IL-18 secretion. Cell Signal 2021;77:109825.

38. Adingupu DD, Gopel SO, Gronros J, et al. SGLT2 inhibition with empagliflozin improves coronary microvascular function and cardiac contractility in prediabetic ob/ob(-/-) mice. Cardiovasc Diabetol 2019;18(1):16.

39. Lee DM, Battson ML, Jarrell DK, et al. SGLT2 inhibition via dapagliflozin improves generalized vascular dysfunction and alters the gut microbiota in type 2 diabetic mice. Cardiovasc Diabetol 2018;17(1):62.

40. Irace C, Cutruzzola A, Parise M, et al. Effect of empagliflozin on brachial artery shear stress and endothelial function in subjects with type 2 diabetes:

Results from an exploratory study. Diab Vasc Dis Res 2020;17(1). 1479164119883540.

41. Sawada T, Uzu K, Hashimoto N, et al. Empagliflozin's ameliorating effect on plasma triglycerides: association with endothelial function recovery in diabetic patients with coronary artery disease. J Atheroscler Thromb 2020;27(7):644–56.

42. Sposito AC, Breder I, Soares AAS, et al. Dapagliflozin effect on endothelial dysfunction in diabetic patients with atherosclerotic disease: a randomized active-controlled trial. Cardiovasc Diabetol 2021;20(1):74.

43. Solini A, Seghieri M, Giannini L, et al. The effects of dapagliflozin on systemic and renal vascular function display an epigenetic signature. J Clin Endocrinol Metab 2019;104(10):4253–63.

44. Zainordin NA, Hatta S, Mohamed Shah FZ, et al. Effects of dapagliflozin on endothelial dysfunction in type 2 diabetes with established ischemic heart disease (EDIFIED). J Endocr Soc 2020;4(1):bvz017.

45. Bosch A, Ott C, Jung S, et al. How does empagliflozin improve arterial stiffness in patients with type 2 diabetes mellitus? Sub analysis of a clinical trial. Cardiovasc Diabetol 2019;18(1):44.

46. Cherney DZ, Perkins BA, Soleymanlou N, et al. The effect of empagliflozin on arterial stiffness and heart rate variability in subjects with uncomplicated type 1 diabetes mellitus. Cardiovasc Diabetol 2014;13:28.

47. Chilton R, Tikkanen I, Cannon CP, et al. Effects of empagliflozin on blood pressure and markers of arterial stiffness and vascular resistance in patients with type 2 diabetes. Diabetes Obes Metab 2015;17(12):1180–93.

48. Hong JY, Park KY, Kim JD, et al. Effects of 6 months of dapagliflozin treatment on metabolic profile and endothelial cell dysfunction for obese type 2 diabetes mellitus patients without atherosclerotic cardiovascular disease. J Obes Metab Syndr 2020;29(3):215–21.

49. Ikonomidis I, Pavlidis G, Thymis J, et al. Effects of glucagon-like peptide-1 receptor agonists, sodium-glucose cotransporter-2 inhibitors, and their combination on endothelial glycocalyx, arterial function, and myocardial work index in patients with type 2 diabetes mellitus after 12-month treatment. J Am Heart Assoc 2020;9(9):e015716.

50. Terasaki M, Hiromura M, Mori Y, et al. Amelioration of hyperglycemia with a sodium-glucose cotransporter 2 inhibitor prevents macrophage-driven atherosclerosis through macrophage foam cell formation suppression in type 1 and type 2 diabetic mice. PLoS One 2015;10(11):e0143396.

51. Dimitriadis GK, Nasiri-Ansari N, Agrogiannis G, et al. Empagliflozin improves primary haemodynamic parameters and attenuates the development of atherosclerosis in high fat diet fed APOE knockout mice. Mol Cell Endocrinol 2019;494:110487.

52. Liu Y, Xu J, Wu M, et al. Empagliflozin protects against atherosclerosis progression by modulating lipid profiles and sympathetic activity. Lipids Health Dis 2021;20(1):5.

53. Chen YC, Jandeleit-Dahm K, Peter K. Sodium-glucose co-transporter 2 (SGLT2) inhibitor dapagliflozin stabilizes diabetes-induced atherosclerotic plaque instability. J Am Heart Assoc 2022;11(1): e022761.

54. D'Onofrio N, Sardu C, Trotta MC, et al. Sodium-glucose co-transporter2 expression and inflammatory activity in diabetic atherosclerotic plaques: Effects of sodium-glucose co-transporter2 inhibitor treatment. Mol Metab 2021;54:101337.

55. Sattar N, McLaren J, Kristensen SL, et al. SGLT2 Inhibition and cardiovascular events: why did EMPA-REG Outcomes surprise and what were the likely mechanisms? Diabetologia 2016;59(7):1333–9.

56. Chiba Y, Yamada T, Tsukita S, et al. Dapagliflozin, a sodium-glucose co-transporter 2 inhibitor, acutely reduces energy expenditure in BAT via neural signals in mice. PLoS One 2016;11(3):e0150756.

57. Elliott RH, Matthews VB, Rudnicka C, et al. Is it time to think about the sodium glucose co-transporter 2 sympathetically? Nephrology (Carlton) 2016;21(4): 286–94.

58. Herat LY, Magno AL, Rudnicka C, et al. SGLT2 inhibitor-induced sympathoinhibition: a novel mechanism for cardiorenal protection. JACC Basic Transl Sci 2020;5(2):169–79.

59. Ridker PM, Everett BM, Thuren T, et al. Antiinflammatory therapy with canakinumab for atherosclerotic disease. N Engl J Med 2017;377(12):1119–31.

60. Bhatt DL, Steg PG, Miller M, et al. Cardiovascular risk reduction with icosapent ethyl for hypertriglyceridemia. N Engl J Med 2019;380(1):11–22.

61. Cannon CP, Blazing MA, Giugliano RP, et al. Ezetimibe added to statin therapy after acute coronary syndromes. N Engl J Med 2015;372(25):2387–97.

SGLT2 Inhibitors and Peripheral Vascular Events
A Review of the Literature

Elena Marchiori, MD[a], Roman N. Rodionov, MD, PhD, FAHA[b,c],
Frederik Peters, PhD[d], Christina Magnussen, MD[e,f],
Joakim Nordanstig, MD, PhD[g], Alexander Gombert, MD[h],
Konstantinos Spanos, MD, PhD[i], Natalia Jarzebska, M.Sc.[b],
Christian-Alexander Behrendt, MD, FESVS[d,j],*

KEYWORDS

- Diabetes • Peripheral arterial disease • SGLT2 inhibitor • Drugs • Outcomes • Amputation

KEY POINTS

- Since first approval of sodium-glucose cotransporter 2 (SGLT2) inhibitors, several randomized controlled trials have shown their benefits for patients with diabetes, heart failure, and kidney disease.
- In 2017, data derived from the CANVAS program suggested a safety signal for canagliflozin in terms of increased lower extremity amputation rates.
- Although the underlying factors, which may influence amputation rates remain unknown to date, the role of a concomitant peripheral arterial disease was discussed.
- This review demonstrated that most studies were not appropriately designed to evaluate peripheral arterial disease (PAD) because only one-fourth of enrolled patients had PAD.

INTRODUCTION

Cardiovascular disease (CVD) has many faces and continues to be the leading cause of death globally. Besides well-known entities such as ischemic heart disease and stroke, people suffering from lower extremity peripheral arterial disease (PAD) are often underrepresented in cardiovascular trials. This anecdotical fact seems striking considering recent epidemiologic data indicating that approximately 237 million people worldwide suffer from intermittent claudication (IC) or chronic limb-threatening ischemia (CLTI).[1–3] In addition, more than 537 million adults between 20 and 79 years are living with diabetes in 2021, thereof many with vascular complications, including PAD.[4,5] Even more disillusioning are the long-term outcomes in the PAD target population.

[a] Department of Vascular and Endovascular Surgery, University Hospital Münster, Münster, Germany; [b] University Center for Vascular Medicine, University Clinic Carl Gustav Carus, Technische Universität Dresden, Germany; [c] College of Medicine and Public Health, Flinders University and Flinders Medical Centre, Adelaide, Australia; [d] Research Group GermanVasc, Department of Vascular Medicine, University Heart and Vascular Center UKE Hamburg, University Medical Center Hamburg-Eppendorf, Hamburg, Germany; [e] Department of Cardiology, University Heart & Vascular Centre Hamburg, Hamburg 20246, Germany; [f] German Centre for Cardiovascular Research (DZHK), Partner Site Hamburg/Kiel/Luebeck, Hamburg, Germany; [g] Institute of Medicine, Department of Molecular and Clinical Medicine, University of Gothenburg and Department of Vascular Surgery, Sahlgrenska University Hospital, Gothenburg, Sweden; [h] European Vascular Centre Aachen-Maastricht, Department of Vascular Surgery, University Hospital RWTH Aachen, Aachen, Germany; [i] Vascular Surgery Department, Larissa University Hospital, Faculty of Medicine, School of Health Sciences, University of Thessaly, Larissa, Greece; [j] Brandenburg Medical School Theodor Fontane, Neuruppin, Germany
* Corresponding author.
E-mail address: behrendt@hamburg.de

Heart Failure Clin 18 (2022) 609–623
https://doi.org/10.1016/j.hfc.2022.03.001
1551-7136/22/© 2022 Elsevier Inc. All rights reserved.

Thirteen to 50% of the patients with IC and 50% to 90% with CLTI will either be dead or suffer from limb loss 5 years after first inpatient treatment.[6,7] In more advanced PAD stages, the prevalence of concomitant chronic kidney disease (CKD) and heart failure can reach almost 30% and 25%, respectively.[8,9] However, the truth is that virtually all patients suffering from PAD face devastating long-term outcomes even before clinically apparent atherosclerosis in other arterial territories has developed. Therefore, recent guidelines suggested that a PAD diagnosis automatically should translate to a "very high risk" label.[10]

During the past decade, the potential benefit of sodium-glucose cotransporter 2 (SGLT2) inhibitors (eg, canagliflozin, dapagliflozin, empagliflozin, ertugliflozin, ipragliflozin, and tofogliflozin) led to a rapid adoption in guidelines primarily addressing patients with heart failure, diabetes, as well as CKD, but not patients with PAD.[11–14] SGLT2 inhibitors exert beneficial effects on cardiac and renal endpoints as well as on other cardiovascular outcomes including overall mortality. Albeit up to 30% of patients with type 2 diabetes also suffer from PAD, to date results from sufficiently powered randomized controlled trials (RCTs) for this subgroup in terms of safety and efficacy are lacking.[15–21] This most recently became an issue when results derived from the CANagliflozin cardioVascular Assessment Study (CANVAS) program (consisting of two sister trials; CANVAS and CANVAS-Renal) led to a heated debate about a safety signal and corresponding warnings about excess amputation rates by national and international regulators (Fig. 1).[18] Strikingly, the emerging safety concerns in 2017 and the subsequent discussions about concomitant PAD as a causative mechanism for the safety signal may have resulted in even lower PAD enrollment rates in trials thereafter. Despite an inherent risk of higher amputation, this target population may benefit substantially from new cardiovascular drugs that target concomitant diabetes, heart failure, and CKD. More than 4 years after the first European Medicines Agency (EMA) and Food and Drug Administration (FDA) pharmacovigilance warning (2017), the debate regarding the potential association with lower extremity amputation persists. This article aims to assess the degree of coverage of PAD patients in existing studies and summarizes the evidence concerning SGLT2 inhibitors and amputation risk.

HISTORY

SGLT2 inhibitors, also known as gliflozins, are derivates of phlorizin, which was first extracted from the bark of apple trees in the nineteenth century.

Almost 2 centuries later, these drugs were first approved by the EMA in April 2012 (dapagliflozin), and by the FDA in March 2013 (canagliflozin). Ever since, 4 different drugs are available for the treatment of type 2 diabetes (2012) and heart failure with reduced ejection fraction (2020).[22–24] On grounds of the unprecedented phase-3 Dapagliflozin And Prevention of Adverse outcomes in Chronic Kidney Disease (DAPA-CKD) trial, the EMA issued a positive opinion and ultimately approved the use of dapagliflozin for the treatment of CKD in August 2021.[25]

AMPUTATION ENDPOINTS AND PERIPHERAL EVENTS IN RANDOMIZED CONTROLLED TRIALS

We provide a review of 18 articles reporting data derived from different RCTs assessing the efficacy and safety of the 6 SGLT2 inhibitors canagliflozin, dapagliflozin, empagliflozin, ertugliflozin, and tofogliflozin (Table 1). Most of these trials assessed dapagliflozin (n = 5, DECLARE-TIMI 58, DAPA-HF, DELIGHT, DAPA-CKD, DERIVE) and 5 empagliflozin (EMPA-REG OUTCOME, EMPEROR-Reduced, EMPEROR-Preserved, and 2 without an acronym),[26,27] 2 trials assessed ertugliflozin (VERTIS SU, VERTIS CV), and 2 assessed canagliflozin (CANVAS Program, CREDENCE). Although most of the trials reported major cardiovascular disease (CVD) prevalence at baseline, PAD data were available only in about half (7 of 15) of trials; 17 articles based on RCT data described amputations in the adverse events discussion. PAD prevalence at baseline varied from 6% to 24%, but in most studies PAD was not highlighted or even analyzed separately. Regarding amputation outcomes, 4 studies reported hazard ratios (HR) for risk difference between SGLT2 inhibitors (canagliflozin, dapagliflozin) and control treatment.[17,28,29] Overall only 7 trials reported both PAD at baseline and data on amputations.

In 2017, the CANVAS program showed that the SGLT2 inhibitor canagliflozin had a beneficial effect on cardiac and renal outcomes. However, the authors also detected a potential safety issue. The CANVAS program involved 10,142 participants in the setting of high cardiovascular risk, including patients with hemodynamically significant PAD and history of amputation secondary to vascular disease. Overall, at baseline 65.6% of the patients had a CVD history and 20.8% a PAD history (see Table 1). Interestingly, 2.3% of the patients had a history of amputation at baseline, and 30.7% a microvascular disease with neuropathy, suggesting the existence of a diabetic foot syndrome. A 2-fold increased risk of lower limb

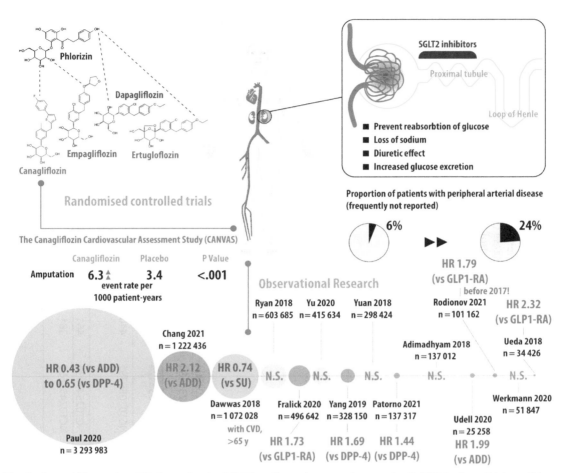

Fig. 1. Central illustration. HR, hazard ratio; SGLT2, sodium-glucose cotransporter 2; DPP-4, dipeptidyl peptidase-4 inhibitors; ADD, antidiabetic drugs; SU, sulfonylurea; CVD, cardiovascular disease; N.S., not significant. Green color denotes an inverse association between SGLT2 inhibitors and amputation (benefit), whereas red color denotes an association between SGLT2 inhibitors and higher amputation rates (harm).

amputation (mostly affecting toes) in the intervention arm (6.3 per 1000 patient-years) compared with placebo (3.4) was observed (HR 1.97; 95% CI 1.41–2.75). Subsequently, a secondary subanalysis further addressed this safety signal and the possible association with differences in the baseline characteristics.[30] Both univariate and multivariate analyses revealed significant associations between amputation at follow-up and baseline risk characteristics including PAD, prior amputation, neuropathy, albuminuria, higher hemoglobin A1c, and random allocation to canagliflozin treatment. Although the overall amputation risk was strongly associated with any history of major or minor amputation and concomitant PAD, the excess amputation risk for canagliflozin users as compared with placebo was similar in each of these subgroups. Furthermore, the risk of amputation was similar for ischemic and infective etiologies and was dose independent.

Conversely to the CANVAS program, the CREDENCE trial that also evaluated canagliflozin reported no significant difference in lower limb amputation risk (HR 1.11; 95% CI 0.79–1.56) and amputation rates of 12.3 (canagliflozin) versus 11.2 (placebo) per 1000 patient-years, whereas there was no difference in baseline characteristics.[17,31]

In 2020, Bonaca and colleagues[28] explicitly determined limb outcomes moderated by history of PAD in the DECLARE-TIMI 58 trial. Patients with concomitant PAD exhibited generally a higher risk of peripheral vascular events, with overall no significant differences between the trial arms (dapagliflozin vs control) regarding adverse ischemic limb events (HR 1.07; 95% CI 0.90–1.26) and amputation (HR 1.09; 95% CI 0.84–1.40). Irrespective of baseline PAD status, dapagliflozin significantly reduced the risk of cardiovascular death and hospitalization for heart failure (with

Table 1
Results of the randomized controlled trials regarding SGLT2 inhibitors in relation to peripheral arterial disease and amputation

Author, Year	Acronym	Drug	NCT	N	Peripheral Arterial Disease (SGLT2i vs Control)	Amputations (SGLT2i vs Control)
Zinman et al,[15] 2015	EMPA-REG OUTCOME	Empagliflozin	NCT01131676	7020	21.0% vs 20.5%	N/A
Neal et al,[29] 2017	CANVAS, CANVAS-R	Canagliflozin	NCT01032629 NCT01989754	10,142	20.8%	6.3 vs 3.4 per 1000 patient-years HR 1.97 (1.41–2.75) no PAD: 5.2 vs 2.4 h 2.34 (1.53–3.58) PAD: 12.1 vs 8.2 h 1.39 (0.80–2.40)
Hollander et al,[19] 2018	VERTIS SU	Ertugliflozin	NCT01999218	1325	N/A	0.1% vs 0.3%
Inzucchi et al,[62] 2018 and Verma et al,[55] 2018	EMPA-REG OUTCOME	Empagliflozin	NCT01131676	7020	21.0% vs 20.5%	1.9% vs 1.8% HR 1.00 (0.70–1.44) no PAD: 0.9% vs 0.7%, HR: 1.30 (0.69–2.46) PAD: 5.5% vs 6.3%, HR: 0.84 (0.54–1.32)
Terauchi et al,[63] 2018	J-STEP/INS	Tofogliflozin	NCT02201004	210	N/A	0 cases
Wiviott et al,[16] 2019	DECLARE-TIMI 58	Dapagliflozin	NCT01730534	17,160	6.0%	1.4% vs 1.3% (P = .53)
McMurray et al,[22] 2019	DAPA-HF	Dapagliflozin	NCT03036124	4744	13.7%	0.5% vs 0.5% (P = 1.00)
Perkovic et al,[17] 2019	CREDENCE	Canagliflozin	NCT02065791	4401#	23.8%	12.3 vs 11.2 per 1000 patient-years HR 1.11 (0.79–1.56)
Pollock et al,[64] 2019	DELIGHT	Dapagliflozin	NCT02547935	461	14%–17% vs 16%	1% vs 0%
Kawamori et al,[26] 2018	N/A	Empagliflozin	NCT02453555	381	N/A	0 cases

Bonaca et al,[28] 2020	DECLARE-TIMI 58	Dapagliflozin	NCT01730534	17,160	6.0%	HR 1.09 (0.84–1.40) no PAD: 0.93 (0.68–1.26) PAD: 1.51 (0.94–2.42)
Cannon et al,[20] 2020	VERTIS CV	Ertugliflozin	NCT01986881	8246	18.7%	2.0% vs 1.6%
Heerspink et al,[25] 2020	DAPA-CKD	Dapagliflozin	NCT03036150	4304#	N/A	1.6% vs 1.8% ($P = .73$)
Packer 2020[23]	EMPEROR-Reduced	Empagliflozin	NCT03057977	3730	N/A	0.7% vs 0.5%
Fioretto 2020[21]	DERIVE	Dapagliflozin	NCT02413398	321	N/A	0 cases
Sone et al,[27] 2020	N/A	Empagliflozin	NCT02589639	269	N/A	0 cases
Anker et al,[24] 2021	EMPEROR-Preserved	Empagliflozin	NCT03057951	5988	N/A	0.5% vs 0.8%

Footnote: #, stopped; HR, hazard ratio; N, number of participants; N/A, not available; NCT, national clinical trial number; RCT, randomized controlled trials; SGLT2i, sodium-glucose cotransporter 2 inhibitors.

Table 2
Results of the meta-analyses regarding SGLT2 inhibitors in relation to peripheral arterial disease and amputation

Author Year	No. of RCTs	Drug	N	Peripheral Arterial Disease	Amputations
Kohler et al,[65] 2017	Pooled Analysis	Empagliflozin	12,620	N/A	1.1 vs 1.1 per 100 patient-years
Rådholm et al,[37] 2018	82	SGLT2i	52,305	N/A	**RR 1.44 (1.13–1.83)[a]**
Li et al,[36] 2018	14	SGLT2i	26,167	N/A	OR 1.40 (0.81–2.41)
Dicembrini et al,[34] 2019	3	SGLT2i	34,322	N/A	OR 1.22 (0.59–2.52)
Zelniker et al,[35] 2019	3	SGLT2i	34,322	N/A	N/A
Yabe et al,[66] 2019	Pooled Analysis	Empagliflozin	2141	N/A	0.0 vs 0.1 per 100 patient-years
Kashiwagi et al,[67] 2019	Pooled Analysis	Ipragliflozin	2005	N/A	0 cases
Tsapas et al,[38] 2020	Pooled Analysis	SGLT2i	93,922	N/A	Canagliflozin **OR 1.61 (1.27–2.05)[a]**
Huang et al,[41] 2020	6	SGLT2i	51,713	N/A	RR 1.24 (0.96–1.60)
Heyward et al,[32] 2020	7	SGLT2i	42,453	N/A	RR 1.28 (0.93–1.76)
Miyashita et al,[39] 2020	5	SGLT2i	39,067	N/A	OR 1.31 (0.92–1.87)
Dorsey-Treviño et al,[68] 2020	3	SGLT2i	31,674	N/A	RR 1.30 (0.93–1.83)
Palmer et al,[40] 2021	764	ADD	421,346	N/A	vs GLP-1: 3.43 (0.14–84.49) vs Thiazolidinedione: 1.13 (0.64–1.99) vs DPP-4: 1.26 (0.86–185) vs placebo: OR 1.14 (0.96–1.35) vs standard therapy: OR 0.38 (0.12–1.20)
Lin et al[33], 2021	39	SGLT2i	74,171	N/A	**OR 1.21 (1.06–1.37)[a]**
Qiu et al,[69] 2021	8	SGLT2i	59,692	N/A	RR 1.21 (0.97–1.51)
McGuire et al,[70] 2021	6	SGLT2i	46,969	N/A	N/A

Footnote: ADD, antidiabetic-drugs; N, number of participants; N/A, not available; No., number; RCT, randomized controlled trial; RR, relative risk; SGLT2i, sodium-glucose cotransporter-2 inhibitors; vs, versus; OR, odds ratio.
[a] Denotes significant values in bold.

PAD: HR 0.86; without PAD: HR 0.82; P-interaction = 0.79) and progression of chronic kidney disease (with PAD: HR 0.78; without PAD: HR 0.76; P-interaction = 0.84).

In recent meta-analyses, the association between amputation and use of SGLT2 inhibitors seem to be restricted to canagliflozin. Although canagliflozin remains the primarily prescribed drug in the United States, dapagliflozin was predominantly used in many European countries. Interestingly, in 11 out of 16 meta-analyses on RCTs, SGLT2 inhibitors were not significantly associated with amputation risk (**Table 2**).

In 7 of 15 articles, drug-specific meta-analyses indicated an increased risk of amputation associated with the use of canagliflozin.[32–38] Rådholm and colleagues[37] (2018) analyzed the available data regarding lower extremity amputation (for canagliflozin and empagliflozin) and described an association of increased risk (relative risk, RR 1.44; 95% CI 1.13–1.83) with a high likelihood of differences between the 2 drugs. In particular, the amputation risk seemed to be restricted to canagliflozin. Concerning patients receiving metformin-based background therapy, Tsapas and colleagues[38] described no increased risk of amputation for patients at low cardiovascular risk and increased amputation risk for patients at high cardiovascular risk in therapy with canagliflozin (OR 1.61; 95% CI 1.27–2.05), under the acknowledgment that the confidence in effect estimates was low. They reported that in drug-naive patients, this analysis for amputation was not performed because of a paucity of pertinent data. Li and colleagues[36] reported that canagliflozin may be positively associated with an increased risk of amputation (OR 1.89; 95% CI 1.37–2.60), compared with oral antidiabetic drugs and placebo, but not empagliflozin (OR 1.02; 95% CI 0.71–1.48), whereas Miyashita and colleagues described that SGLT2 inhibitors were not associated with a significantly increased risk of amputation compared with controls (OR 1.31; 95% CI 0.92–1.87). Their subgroup meta-analysis demonstrated that neither canagliflozin (OR 1.60; 95% CI 0.79–3.26) nor empagliflozin (OR 1.03; 95% CI 0.72–1.49) or dapagliflozin were associated with increased risk of amputation.[39]

In an extensive systematic review and network meta-analysis of 764 trials assessing 2 drug classes (SGLT2 inhibitors and GLP1-RA; glucagon-like peptide-1 receptor agonists) on the top of the existing diabetes therapy, Palmer and colleagues[40] assessed the odds for amputations with SGLT2 inhibitors compared with other treatments and placebo. This analysis did not show any significantly increased risk for SGLT2 inhibitors as a class with any of the other treatments. The authors reported odds for SGLT2 inhibitors versus GLP1-RA of 3.43 (95% CI 0.14–84.49), versus thiazolidinedione 1.13 (95% CI 0.64–1.99), versus dipeptidyl-peptidase-4 (DPP-4) inhibitors 1.26 (95% CI 0.86–1.85), versus standard therapy 0.38 (95% CI 0.12–1.20), and versus placebo 1.14 (95% CI 0.96–1.35). Their network plot for amputation emphasized the paucity of head-to head trials comparing amputation outcomes between different treatments.

In 2020 Huang and colleagues[41] performed a meta-analysis of 6 large RCTs reporting overall no increased risk of lower-limb amputations related to SGLT-2 inhibitors; importantly this conclusion endured also in subgroup analyses regarding PAD. They propose that amputation events would mainly arise from chronic limb-threatening ischemia and infection instead of acute limb ischemia. More recently, some meta-analyses addressed the issue of incident PAD in RCTs. Li and colleagues[36] reported a significantly higher incidence of a PAD with SGLT2 inhibitors (OR 1.21; 95% CI 1.03–1.42; P = .02), whereas Dicembrini and colleagues reported an overall lower incidence (OR 1.26; 95% CI 1.04, 1.52). A subgroup analysis of the latter showed significantly increased risk only with canagliflozin and a significant reduction of risk with empagliflozin.[34]

Overall, there is no consistent high-level evidence suggesting that SGLT2 inhibitor exposure independently leads to an increased risk of amputation. The effects of medical treatment on amputation risk could substantially vary based on the baseline cardiovascular and renal risk profile. Moreover, certainly, the patient selection and prescription practice may also differ widely, especially in patients enrolled after the 2017 EMA and FDA warnings. Two major aspects limit the understanding of the interplay of PAD and amputations while on SGLT2 treatment in trials on SGLT2 inhibitors. First, as **Table 1** illustrates, in most RCTs, the PAD prevalence and disease stage was not assessed and consistently reported as prespecified baseline parameters, although eligibility criteria comprised established atherosclerotic cardiovascular disease (including PAD manifestations). Second, the severity and cause of the limb events was rarely reported.

OBSERVATIONAL STUDIES COMPARING SGLT2 INHIBITORS WITH OTHER TREATMENTS

Results from observational data investigating the impact of SGLT2 inhibitors on lower limb outcome report conflicting findings and conclusions as well. Sixteen observational studies with cohorts accounting 25,258 to 3,293,983 patients were evaluated (**Table 3**). Twelve reported PAD data at baseline and all 16 statistically compared amputation outcomes between SGLT2 inhibitors and other antidiabetic-drugs (ADD). Three population-based studies specifically assessed the risk of amputation with canagliflozin, thereof 2 reporting no significantly increased risk of amputation and one reporting an increased risk restricted to the subgroup of patients with CVD and age greater than 65 years.[42–44] In this subgroup, the prevalence of PAD was 21.3% at baseline. In opposite to the previously cited RCTs and meta-analyses, Yuan and colleagues[43] analyzed a health claims database to determine the incidence of below the knee (BTK) amputation in new users of canagliflozin versus non-SGLT2 inhibitors (118,018 vs 226,623 patients). This study revealed no evidence suggesting an increased risk (1.18 vs 1.12 events per 1000 person-years; HR 0.98; 95% CI 0.68–1.41). Ryan and colleagues[42] performed a large comprehensive analysis using data from 4 large United States administrative claims databases including patients who were treated with canagliflozin. The authors stated consistent benefits regarding the risk of hospitalization for heart failure with no increased risk of amputation (HR 0.75; 95% CI 0.40–1.41 on treatment; HR 1.01; 95%

Table 3
Results of the observational studies regarding SGLT2 inhibitors in relation to peripheral arterial disease and amputation

Author Year	Drug	Comparator	N	Patient Subgroups	Peripheral Arterial Disease	Amputation Risk
Udell et al,[71] 2017	SGLT2i	ADD	25,258	N/A	16% SGLT2i 20.4% non-SGLT2i	**HR 1.99 (1.12–3.51)**[a]
Dawwas [52] 2018	SGLT2i	SU DPP-4	1,072,028	N/A	N/A	vs SU: **HR 0.74 (0.57–0.96)**[a] vs DPP-4: HR 0.88 (0.65–1.15)
Ryan et al,[42] 2018	Canagliflozin	ADD	603,685	N/A	N/A	on treatment: HR 0.75 (0.40–1.41) intent-to-treat: HR 1.01 (0.93–1.10)
Yuan et al,[43] 2018	Canagliflozin	ADD	298,424	N/A	8.5% canagliflozin 8.6% ADD	HR 0.98 (0.68–1.41)
Adimadhyam et al,[72] 2018	SGLT2i	DPP-4	137,012	N/A	4.5% overall 4.61% SGLT2i 4.34% DPP-4	HR 1.38 (0.83–2.31)
Ueda et al,[47] 2018	SGLT2i	GLP1-RA	34,426	N/A	6% overall	**HR 2.32 (1.37–3.91)**[a]
Chang et al,[46] 2018	SGLT2i	DPP-4 GLP-1 ADD	953,906	N/A	N/A	vs DPP-4: HR 1.50 (0.85–2.67) vs GLP-1: HR 1.47 (0.64–3.36) vs ADD: **HR 2.12 (1.19–3.77)**[a]
Yang et al,[48] 2019	SGLT2i	DPP-4 SU	328,150	N/A	2.8% SGLT2i 2.8% DPP-4 2.2% SU	vs DPP-4: **HR 1.69 (1.20–2.38)**[a] vs SU: HR 1.02 (0.54–1.93)
Paul [50] 2020	SGLT2i	GLP1-RA DPP-4 ADD	3,293,983	N/A	6% SGLT2i 4% GLP1-RA 6% DPP-4 5% others ADD	vs GLP1-RA: HR 0.88 (0.73–1.05) vs DPP-4: HR 0.65 (0.56–0.75)[a] vs ADD: **HR 0.43 (0.37–0.49)**[a]

Study	Drug	Comparator	N	Subgroup	%	HR (CI)
Fralick et al,[44] 2020	Canagliflozin	GLP1-RA	496,642	with CVD <65 y	19.6% canagliflozin 19.3% GLP1-RA	HR 1.18 (0.86–1.62)
				with CVD >65 y	21.3% canagliflozin 21.1% GLP1-RA	**HR 1.73 (1.30–2.29)[a]**
				no CVD <65 y	0% overall	HR 1.09 (0.83–1.43)
				no CVD >65 y	0% overall	HR 1.30 (0.52–3.26)
Yu et al,[73] 2020	SGLT2i	DPP-4	415,634	N/A	2.2% SGLT2i 2.2% DPP-4	HR 0.88 (0.71–1.09)
Udell et al,[74] 2020	Canagliflozin	ADD	110,229	N/A	15.4% canagliflozin 20.2% non-SGLT2i	HR 1.44 (0.82–2.52)
Werkman et al,[75] 2020	SGLT2i	SU	51,847	N/A	1.5% SGLT2i 1.9% SU	HR 0.70 (0.38–1.29)
Chang et al,[53] 2021	SGLT2i	DPP-4 GLP1-RA ADD	1,222,436	N/A	N/A	vs DPP-4: HR 0.38 (0.04–3.73) vs GLP1-RA: N/A vs ADD: HR 0.61 (0.05–7.36)
Patorno et al,[49] 2021	SGLT2i	GLP1-RA	137,317	N/A	12.4% SGLT2i 13.7% GLP1-RA	**HR 1.44 (1.06–1.96)[a]**
Rodionov et al,[54] 2021	SGLT2i	GLP1-RA	101,162	Without PAD	0% overall	Before EMA warning: HR 1.79 (1.03–3.02)[a] after EMA warning: HR 0.89 (0.57–1.33)
				With PAD	13.6% SGLT2i 16.3% GLP1-RA	Before EMA warning: HR 1.31 (0.89–1.87) after EMA warning: HR 1.24 (0.84–1.77)

Footnote: ADD, other antidiabetic-drugs; CVD, cardiovascular disease; DPP-4, dipeptidyl peptidase-4 inhibitors; EMA, European medicines agency; GLP1-RA, glucagon-like peptide-1 receptor agonist; HR, hazard ratio; N, number of participants; N/A, not available; PAD, peripheral arterial disease; SGLT2i, sodium-glucose cotransporter 2 inhibitors; SU, sulfonylurea.
[a] Denotes significant values in bold.

CI 0.93–1.10 intent-to-treat). These results persisted in the subpopulation with established cardiovascular disease.

Scrutinizing SGLT2 inhibitors as a class, overall, in 7 of 14 observational studies SGLT2 inhibitors were in some form significantly associated with amputation risk (see **Table 3**). Based on matched health insurance claims data from patients enrolled in one of the largest public programs in the United States, Udell and colleagues[45] reported a 2-fold higher risk for lower-limb amputation in patients initiating SGLT2i at baseline (58.1% canagliflozin, 26.4% empagliflozin, and 15.5% dapagliflozin) as compared with those initiating other antihyperglycemic agents. A roughly similar finding was reported by Chang and colleagues[46] 2018, where SGLTi users had a higher amputation risk than users of other antidiabetic drugs (HR 2.12; 95% CI 1.19–3.77) but not in comparison with DPP-4 (HR 1.50; 95% CI 0.85–2.67) and GLP-1 (HR 1.47, 95% CI 0.64–3.36).

Use of SGLT2 inhibitors was significantly associated with an increased risk of lower-limb amputation in a propensity score matched European cohort by Ueda and colleagues[47] with GLP1-RA as active comparator (HR 2.32; 95% CI 1.37–3.91). These results were confirmed in an analysis by Yang and colleagues[48] with a significant association using DPP-4 as active comparator (HR 1.69; 95% CI 1.20–2.38) but not sulfonylurea (HR 1.02; 95% CI 0.54–1.93). Fralick and colleagues[44] documented a higher amputation risk in patients older than 65 and baseline cardiovascular disease but not in younger patients and those without baseline cardiovascular disease. Similarly, using Medicare data focusing on patients older than 65 years, Patorno and colleagues[49] reported a 44% higher risk for lower-limb amputation (HR 1.44; 95% CI 1.06–1.96) irrespective of a history of cardiovascular disease.

On the contrary, Paul and colleagues[50] applied a propensity score-matched observational study design to demonstrate a protective effect of SGLT2 inhibitors in terms of lower risk of amputation using either DPP-4 (HR 0.65; 95% CI 0.56–0.75) or other antidiabetic drugs (HR 0.43; 95% CI 0.37–0.49) as active comparator. This study revealed similar rates of amputation with canagliflozin, empagliflozin, and dapagliflozin. Of note, the groups in this study were not clearly distinct because patients taking SLGT2 inhibitors were allowed to also be treated with GLP-1 or DPP-4.[51]

Using databases from the United States, Dawwas and colleagues[52] reported that SGLT2 inhibitors as a class decreased the risk of developing incident cardiovascular disease. Furthermore, the amputation risk in the comparison with DPP-4 (HR 0.88; 95% CI 0.65–1.15) as well as with sulfonylureas (HR 0.74; 95% CI 0.57–0.96) decreased.

In 2021, Chang and colleagues published a retrospective study analyzing new users of SGTL2 inhibitors in the Taiwan National Health Insurance Database.[53] Limb outcomes included lower extremity amputation, PAD, and critical limb ischemia (CLI). For this study, 2 cohorts were sampled. A first cohort, which excluded patients with baseline history of amputation (n = 1,222,436), was used to evaluate amputation outcomes while only 8200 patients with SGLT2 inhibitor therapy and 1700 patients with GLP1-RA were included and only one amputation event occurred after 1 year. No significant differences concerning the risk of lower extremity amputation across medication groups, and new use of SGLT2 inhibitors were observed for different active comparators including DPP-4 (HR 0.38; 95% CI 0.04–3.73) and ADD (HR 0.61; 95% CI 0.05–7.36). The incidence rate of amputation per 10,000 person-years amounted to 1.5, 4.6, 6.1, and 1.9 for SGLT2 inhibitors, DPP-4, GLP1-RA, and ADD, respectively. In a second cohort excluding patients with history of amputation, PAD, and CLI at baseline, new use of SGLT2 inhibitors was significantly associated with incident PAD compared with new users of GLP1-RA (HR, 1.47; 95% CI 1.03–2.09), whereas there was no significant risk with other ADD comparators. Moreover, the study concluded that SGLT2 inhibitors were associated with lower mortality compared with DPP-4 inhibitors.

Recently, our research group used nationwide health insurance claims from Germany including more than 100,000 patients with diabetes to compare new use of SGLT2 inhibitors with GLP1-RA as active comparator.[54] The study confirmed that patients with diabetes and PAD have considerable high risk of amputations in the longer term. Periods before and after the EMA warning in 2017 were analyzed separately and stratified by the presence of concomitant PAD. Before the EMA warning, initiation of SGLT2 inhibitors was associated with a lower risk of hospitalization for heart failure in patients with PAD (HR 0.85; 95% CI 0.73–0.99) and a higher risk of lower extremity amputation in patients without PAD (HR 1.79; 95% CI 1.04–2.92). After the EMA warning, however, the efficacy and safety endpoints were no longer statistically different between groups what emphasized that the prescription practice may have changed.

In conclusion, there was no consistent evidence of an increased risk of peripheral vascular events and amputations in observational studies. The main limitation in the comparison between observational studies is the inconsistent and imprecise definition of amputation and the paucity of data regarding the PAD stage. Moreover, it is possible that an allocation bias occurred, due to the ongoing debate and safety issues regarding amputation risks with SGLT2 inhibitors.

METHODOLOGICAL CONSIDERATIONS

From a methodological standpoint, a well-balanced assessment of the actual amputation risk associated with the use of SGLT2 inhibitors seems challenging if not impossible. To date, the most solid evidence on the matter rests on the results from the CANVAS program. Here, the potential amputation risk was not captured systematically before the final months of the trial, whereas earlier events were documented less strict through the adverse events reporting. In EMPA-REG OUTCOME, completed 2 years before the publication of the CANVAS findings, amputations were later identified less reliable partly from adverse event reporting and partly from narratives, case report forms, or in investigator comments.[55] In response to the reported elevated amputation risk and associated warnings from official bodies, CREDENCE amended its protocol to ask investigators to interrupt treatment in case of foot complications.[17] Similarly, amputations were not prespecified adverse events in DECLARE-TIMI 58, but started to be collected retrospectively and prospectively during the study in response to the warnings.[16] Thus, for these large earlier trials, it is unknown to which extent the initially unspecified collection of amputations affected the final results. Yet, later trials such as EMPEROR-Preserved that did assess this endpoint systematically did also not confirm the safety signal.[24]

Doubtless, the CANVAS results dominated the central estimates of the meta-analyses, especially those focusing on canagliflozin.

A big advantage of observational studies is the somewhat more objective retrospective assessment of amputations through electronic health records. However, at the same time, these studies suffer from the lack of randomization and the lack of a placebo group. In fact, all amputation risk estimates for SGLT2 inhibitors in this group of studies rest on the main assumption that these patients are comparable to those taking other antidiabetic agents, at least after adjustment for observed confounding. Besides, the design of observational studies is more vulnerable to biases related to the timing of initiation of the treatment and treatment history.[56] Moreover, the follow-up time of these analyses is often too short for detecting a sufficient number of outcomes occurring rarely and late.[51]

DISCUSSION

The current review identified 18 RCTs evaluating the safety and effectiveness of SGLT2 inhibitors in patients with diabetes, heart failure, and CKD. Although most of the included trials were not primarily designed and powered to determine lower extremity amputations as an outcome, only 7 reported PAD status at baseline. Except for the CANVAS program, which enrolled patients treated with canagliflozin, no other RCT or any drug in this class reported significantly higher amputation rates in patients who were treated with SGLT2 inhibitors. This inconsistency of evidence was further emphasized by conflicting conclusions derived from several observational cohort studies with varying methods. Despite all that, the unique CANVAS data on excess amputation risk led to a heated international debate and numerous regulatory warnings concerning the safety of these drugs involving large cardiovascular disease populations. It is not unlikely that this tentative safety issue withheld the use of these important cardiovascular-protective compounds in the specific setting of PAD with type 2 diabetes, despite the well-established very-high cardiovascular risk in this patient population.

During the past years, various hypotheses have been generated to explain this safety signal. Potier and colleagues[57] have recently commented on a possible volume depletion effect of SGLT2 inhibitors causing lower limb complications. Supporting this hypothesis, Lin and colleagues recently conducted a meta-analysis of 39 RCTs (thereof 15 included in a meta-analysis on amputation risk) and found that the risk of amputation was slightly increased in patients with canagliflozin treatment but not in patients treated with other SGLT2 inhibitors. Furthermore, reductions in body weight and blood pressure were associated with those complications, lending support to a hemodynamic hypothesis where both PAD and amputation may be triggered (or unmasked) by the well-known initial effects on body fluid composition when initiating SGLT2 inhibitors. Overall, the OR was 1.23 (95% CI 1.08–1.40) with 599 events in the SGLT2 group versus 369 among controls.[33] Also emphasizing this volume hypothesis, previous studies showed that there was a trend toward higher event rates in patients treated with diuretics.[58–60] Sherman and colleagues (2018) recently evaluated the impact of canagliflozin on blood flow recovery in a murine surrogate model. Interestingly, contrary to the initial study hypothesis, the results suggested that canagliflozin administration did not impair the efficiency of endogenous vascular recovery.[61] Hence, the underlying role of hypovolemia should be specifically assessed clinically or via biochemical markers in future studies with SGLT2 inhibitors to further investigate the effect of this potential confounder on the outcomes of interest.

Due to the obvious association between PAD and amputation, it was further hypothesized that the events may only occur in the subgroup with any history of PAD. Hence, several recruiting trials have subsequently adapted their enrollment and surveillance strategies in line with issued regulatory warnings. This in turn makes it very challenging to validly assess the safety of SGLT2 inhibitors because participants at higher risk for suffering the endpoint of interest (ie, amputation) may have been excluded from trial participation.

To further determine both the underlying factors driving lower extremity amputation in patients treated with SGLT2 inhibitors as well as the hypothesized changes in patient selection, our research group recently conducted a retrospective analysis of more than 100,000 patients with diabetes and PAD who were treated between 2013 and 2019 to compare outcomes in patients treated with SGLT2 inhibitors versus GLP1-RAs as active comparator. Periods before and after the EMA warning were analyzed separately and stratified by the presence of concomitant PAD. The fact that excess amputation rates were only observed in diabetics without concomitant PAD refuted the idea that the presence of PAD explained the excess amputation risk. Certainly, patients with PAD benefit from SGLT2 inhibitors in terms of lower hospitalization rates for heart failure. Also interesting, all differentials—both benefits and harms—among study groups diminished after the regulatory warning in 2017 emphasizing that prescription practices changed.[54]

SUMMARY

The current review on amputation rates in trials and observational research on SGLT2 inhibitor therapy emphasized that the very-low proportion of included PAD patients, the heterogeneity of methods as well as the lack of precise data on baseline PAD status and amputation endpoints impede the generation of a careful conclusion. Less than one-fourth of recent cohorts had PAD and many trials were not designed to evaluate the relationship between SGLT2 inhibitors and amputation rates either. Only the CANVAS program evaluating canagliflozin suggested a safety signal, whereas conclusions from studies using real-world data were inconsistent. Although the safety signal in the CANVAS program was picked up based on routine adverse event data collection, subsequent trials were enforced by regulators to consider amputations as adverse event of special interest, which may have led to more complete and granular data based on adjudication by independent committees.

CLINICS CARE POINTS

- RCTs on SGLT2 inhibitors were not primarily powered to determine the interaction between PAD, SGLT2 inhibitor therapy, and lower extremity amputations as an outcome
- The CANVAS program and a secondary analysis of trial data revealed a significant association between canagliflozin and lower extremity amputation rate during follow-up
- There is no consistent evidence that SGLT2 inhibitors as a drug class increase peripheral vascular events and lower extremity amputations in the longer term
- Future research and trials on pharmacotherapy of cardiovascular disease shall consider adjusting the design to better cover patients with PAD

DISCLOSURE

The authors have no conflicts of interest.

REFERENCES

1. Song P, Rudan D, Zhu Y, et al. Global, regional, and national prevalence and risk factors for peripheral artery disease in 2015: an updated systematic review and analysis. Lancet Glob Health 2019;7(8): e1020–30.
2. Fowkes FG, Rudan D, Rudan I, et al. Comparison of global estimates of prevalence and risk factors for peripheral artery disease in 2000 and 2010: a systematic review and analysis. Lancet 2013; 382(9901):1329–40.
3. Chen Q, Li L, Chen Q, et al. Critical appraisal of international guidelines for the screening and treatment of asymptomatic peripheral artery disease: a systematic review. BMC Cardiovasc Disord 2019; 19(1):17.
4. IDF diabetes atlas, 10th edition., Brussels, Belgium. 2021. Available at: https://www.diabetesatlas.org. Accessed 30th Nov 2021.

5. Stoberock K, Kaschwich M, Nicolay SS, et al. The interrelationship between diabetes mellitus and peripheral arterial disease. VASA 2021;50(5):323–30.

6. Kreutzburg T, Peters F, Kuchenbecker J, et al. Editor's choice - the germanvasc score: a pragmatic risk score predicts five year amputation free survival in patients with peripheral arterial occlusive disease. Eur J Vasc Endovasc Surg 2021;61(2):248–56.

7. Baubeta Fridh E, Andersson M, Thuresson M, et al. Amputation rates, mortality, and pre-operative comorbidities in patients revascularised for intermittent claudication or critical limb ischaemia: a population based study. Eur J Vasc Endovasc Surg 2017; 54(4):480–6.

8. Kotov A, Peters F, Debus ES, et al. The prospective GermanVasc cohort study. VASA Z Gefasskrankheiten 2021;50(6):446–52.

9. Kreutzburg T, Peters F, Riess HC, et al. Editor's choice - comorbidity patterns among patients with peripheral arterial occlusive disease in germany: a trend analysis of health insurance claims data. Eur J Vasc Endovasc Surg 2020;59(1):59–66.

10. Mach F, Baigent C, Catapano AL, et al. 2019 ESC/EAS Guidelines for the management of dyslipidaemias: lipid modification to reduce cardiovascular risk. Eur Heart J 2020;41(1):111–88.

11. McDonagh TA, Metra M, Adamo M, et al. 2021 ESC Guidelines for the diagnosis and treatment of acute and chronic heart failure. Eur Heart J 2021;42(36): 3599–726.

12. Visseren FLJ, Mach F, Smulders YM, et al. 2021 ESC Guidelines on cardiovascular disease prevention in clinical practice. Eur Heart J 2021;42(34):3227–337.

13. Cosentino F, Grant PJ, Aboyans V, et al. 2019 ESC Guidelines on diabetes, pre-diabetes, and cardiovascular diseases developed in collaboration with the EASD. Eur Heart J 2020;41(2):255–323.

14. American Diabetes A. 9. Pharmacologic approaches to glycemic treatment: standards of medical care in diabetes-2021. Diabetes Care 2021; 44(Suppl 1):S111–24.

15. Zinman B, Wanner C, Lachin JM, et al. Empagliflozin, cardiovascular outcomes, and mortality in type 2 diabetes. N Engl J Med 2015;373(22):2117–28.

16. Wiviott SD, Raz I, Bonaca MP, et al. Dapagliflozin and cardiovascular outcomes in type 2 diabetes. N Engl J Med 2019;380(4):347–57.

17. Perkovic V, Jardine MJ, Neal B, et al. Canagliflozin and renal outcomes in type 2 diabetes and nephropathy. N Engl J Med 2019;380(24):2295–306.

18. Neal B, Perkovic V, Matthews DR. Canagliflozin and cardiovascular and renal events in type 2 diabetes. N Engl J Med 2017;377(21):2099.

19. Hollander P, Liu J, Hill J, et al. Ertugliflozin compared with glimepiride in patients with type 2 diabetes mellitus inadequately controlled on metformin: the VERTIS SU randomized study. Diabetes Ther 2018; 9(1):193–207.

20. Cannon CP, Pratley R, Dagogo-Jack S, et al. Cardiovascular outcomes with ertugliflozin in type 2 diabetes. N Engl J Med 2020;383(15):1425–35.

21. Fioretto P, Del Prato S, Buse JB, et al. Efficacy and safety of dapagliflozin in patients with type 2 diabetes and moderate renal impairment (chronic kidney disease stage 3A): The DERIVE Study. Diabetes Obes Metab 2018;20(11):2532–40.

22. McMurray JJV, Solomon SD, Inzucchi SE, et al. Dapagliflozin in patients with heart failure and reduced ejection fraction. N Engl J Med 2019;381(21): 1995–2008.

23. Packer M, Anker SD, Butler J, et al. Cardiovascular and renal outcomes with empagliflozin in heart failure. N Engl J Med 2020;383(15):1413–24.

24. Anker SD, Butler J, Filippatos G, et al. Empagliflozin in heart failure with a preserved ejection fraction. N Engl J Med 2021;385(16):1451–61.

25. Heerspink HJL, Stefánsson BV, Correa-Rotter R, et al. Dapagliflozin in patients with chronic kidney disease. N Engl J Med 2020;383(15):1436–46.

26. Kawamori R, Haneda M, Suzaki K, et al. Empagliflozin as add-on to linagliptin in a fixed-dose combination in Japanese patients with type 2 diabetes: Glycaemic efficacy and safety profile in a 52-week, randomized, placebo-controlled trial. Diabetes Obes Metab 2018;20(9):2200–9.

27. Sone H, Kaneko T, Shiki K, et al. Efficacy and safety of empagliflozin as add-on to insulin in Japanese patients with type 2 diabetes: a randomized, double-blind, placebo-controlled trial. Diabetes Obes Metab 2020;22(3):417–26.

28. Bonaca MP, Wiviott SD, Zelniker TA, et al. Dapagliflozin and cardiac, kidney, and limb outcomes in patients with and without peripheral artery disease in DECLARE-TIMI 58. Circulation 2020;142(8):734–47.

29. Neal B, Perkovic V, Mahaffey KW, et al. Canagliflozin and cardiovascular and renal events in type 2 diabetes. N Engl J Med 2017;377(7):644–57.

30. Matthews DR, Li Q, Perkovic V, et al. Effects of canagliflozin on amputation risk in type 2 diabetes: the CANVAS program. Diabetologia 2019;62(6):926–38.

31. Arnott C, Huang Y, Neuen BL, et al. The effect of canagliflozin on amputation risk in the CANVAS program and the CREDENCE trial. Diabetes Obes Metab 2020;22(10):1753–66.

32. Heyward J, Mansour O, Olson L, et al. Association between sodium-glucose cotransporter 2 (SGLT2) inhibitors and lower extremity amputation: a systematic review and meta-analysis. PLoS one 2020;15(6): e0234065.

33. Lin C, Zhu X, Cai X, et al. SGLT2 inhibitors and lower limb complications: an updated meta-analysis. Cardiovasc Diabetol. 2021;20(1):91.

34. Dicembrini I, Tomberli B, Nreu B, et al. Peripheral artery disease and amputations with Sodium-Glucose co-Transporter-2 (SGLT-2) inhibitors: A meta-analysis of randomized controlled trials. Diabetes Res Clin Pract 2019;153:138–44.

35. Zelniker TA, Wiviott SD, Raz I, et al. SGLT2 inhibitors for primary and secondary prevention of cardiovascular and renal outcomes in type 2 diabetes: a systematic review and meta-analysis of cardiovascular outcome trials. Lancet 2019;393(10166):31–9.

36. Li D, Yang JY, Wang T, et al. Risks of diabetic foot syndrome and amputation associated with sodium glucose co-transporter 2 inhibitors: a meta-analysis of randomized controlled trials. Diabetes Metab 2018;44(5):410–4.

37. Rådholm K, Wu JH, Wong MG, et al. Effects of sodium-glucose cotransporter-2 inhibitors on cardiovascular disease, death and safety outcomes in type 2 diabetes - A systematic review. Diabetes Res Clin Pract 2018;140:118–28.

38. Tsapas A, Avgerinos I, Karagiannis T, et al. Comparative effectiveness of glucose-lowering drugs for type 2 diabetes: a systematic review and network meta-analysis. Ann Intern Med 2020;173(4):278–86.

39. Miyashita S, Kuno T, Takagi H, et al. Risk of amputation associated with sodium-glucose co-transporter 2 inhibitors: a meta-analysis of five randomized controlled trials. Diabetes Res Clin Pract 2020;163:108136.

40. Palmer SC, Tendal B, Mustafa RA, et al. Sodium-glucose cotransporter protein-2 (SGLT-2) inhibitors and glucagon-like peptide-1 (GLP-1) receptor agonists for type 2 diabetes: systematic review and network meta-analysis of randomised controlled trials. BMJ 2021;372:m4573.

41. Huang CY, Lee JK. Sodium-glucose co-transporter-2 inhibitors and major adverse limb events: a trial-level meta-analysis including 51 713 individuals. Diabetes Obes Metab 2020;22(12):2348–55.

42. Ryan PB, Buse JB, Schuemie MJ, et al. Comparative effectiveness of canagliflozin, SGLT2 inhibitors and non-SGLT2 inhibitors on the risk of hospitalization for heart failure and amputation in patients with type 2 diabetes mellitus: a real-world meta-analysis of 4 observational databases (OBSERVE-4D). Diabetes Obes Metab 2018;20(11):2585–97.

43. Yuan Z, DeFalco FJ, Ryan PB, et al. Risk of lower extremity amputations in people with type 2 diabetes mellitus treated with sodium-glucose co-transporter-2 inhibitors in the USA: a retrospective cohort study. Diabetes Obes Metab 2018;20(3):582–9.

44. Fralick M, Kim SC, Schneeweiss S, et al. Risk of amputation with canagliflozin across categories of age and cardiovascular risk in three US nationwide databases: cohort study. BMJ 2020;370:m2812.

45. Udell JA, Yuan Z, Rush T, et al. Cardiovascular outcomes and risks after initiation of a sodium glucose cotransporter 2 inhibitor: results from the EASEL population-based cohort study (evidence for cardiovascular outcomes with sodium glucose cotransporter 2 inhibitors in the real world). Circulation 2018;137(14):1450–9.

46. Chang HY, Singh S, Mansour O, et al. Association between sodium-glucose cotransporter 2 inhibitors and lower extremity amputation among patients with type 2 diabetes. JAMA Intern Med 2018;178(9):1190–8.

47. Ueda P, Svanström H, Melbye M, et al. Sodium glucose cotransporter 2 inhibitors and risk of serious adverse events: nationwide register based cohort study. BMJ 2018;363:k4365.

48. Yang JY, Wang T, Pate V, et al. Sodium-glucose cotransporter-2 inhibitor use and risk of lower-extremity amputation: evolving questions, evolving answers. Diabetes Obes Metab 2019;21(5):1223–36.

49. Patorno E, Pawar A, Bessette LG, et al. Comparative effectiveness and safety of sodium-glucose cotransporter 2 inhibitors versus glucagon-like peptide 1 receptor agonists in older adults. Diabetes Care 2021;44(3):826–35.

50. Paul SK, Bhatt DL, Montvida O. The association of amputations and peripheral artery disease in patients with type 2 diabetes mellitus receiving sodium-glucose cotransporter type-2 inhibitors: real-world study. Eur Heart J 2021;42(18):1728–38.

51. Vlachopoulos C, Terentes-Printzios D, Tsioufis K. Do SGLT2 inhibitors increase the risk of amputation? Make haste slowly. Eur Heart J 2021;42(18):1739–41.

52. Dawwas GK, Smith SM, Park H. Cardiovascular outcomes of sodium glucose cotransporter-2 inhibitors in patients with type 2 diabetes. Diabetes Obes Metab 2019;21(1):28–36.

53. Chang HY, Chou YY, Tang W, et al. Association of antidiabetic therapies with lower extremity amputation, mortality and healthcare cost from a nationwide retrospective cohort study in Taiwan. Scientific Rep 2021;11(1):7000.

54. Rodionov RN, Peters F, Marschall U, et al. Initiation of SGLT2 inhibitors and the risk of lower extremity minor and major amputation in patients with type 2 diabetes and peripheral arterial disease: a health claims data analysis. Eur J Vasc Endovasc Surg 2021;62(6):981–90.

55. Verma S, Mazer CD, Al-Omran M, et al. Cardiovascular outcomes and safety of empagliflozin in patients with type 2 diabetes mellitus and peripheral artery disease: a subanalysis of EMPA-REG OUTCOME. Circulation 2018;137(4):405–7.

56. Suissa S. Reduced mortality with sodium-glucose cotransporter-2 inhibitors in observational studies: avoiding immortal time bias. Circulation 2018;137(14):1432–4.

57. Potier L, Mohammedi K, Velho G, et al. SGLT2 inhibitors and lower limb complications: the diuretic-induced hypovolemia hypothesis. Cardiovasc Diabetol 2021;20(1):107.

58. Officers A. Coordinators for the ACRGTA, lipid-lowering treatment to prevent heart attack T. Major outcomes in high-risk hypertensive patients randomized to angiotensin-converting enzyme inhibitor or calcium channel blocker vs diuretic: The Antihypertensive and Lipid-Lowering Treatment to Prevent Heart Attack Trial (ALLHAT). JAMA 2002;288(23):2981–97.

59. Brown MJ, Palmer CR, Castaigne A, et al. Morbidity and mortality in patients randomised to double-blind treatment with a long-acting calcium-channel blocker or diuretic in the International Nifedipine GITS study: intervention as a Goal in Hypertension Treatment (INSIGHT). Lancet 2000;356(9227):366–72.

60. Erkens JA, Klungel OH, Stolk RP, et al. Antihypertensive drug therapy and the risk of lower extremity amputations in pharmacologically treated type 2 diabetes patients. Pharmacoepidemiol Drug Saf 2004;13(3):139–46.

61. Sherman SE, Bell GI, Teoh H, et al. Canagliflozin improves the recovery of blood flow in an experimental model of severe limb ischemia. JACC Basic Transl Sci 2018;3(2):327–9.

62. Inzucchi SE, Zinman B, Fitchett D, et al. How does empagliflozin reduce cardiovascular mortality? insights from a mediation analysis of the EMPA-REG OUTCOME trial. Diabetes Care 2018;41(2):356–63.

63. Terauchi Y, Tamura M, Senda M, et al. Long-term safety and efficacy of tofogliflozin as add-on to insulin in patients with type 2 diabetes: Results from a 52-week, multicentre, randomized, double-blind, open-label extension, Phase 4 study in Japan (J-STEP/INS). Diabetes Obes Metab 2018;20(5):1176–85.

64. Pollock C, Stefansson B, Reyner D, et al. Albuminuria-lowering effect of dapagliflozin alone and in combination with saxagliptin and effect of dapagliflozin and saxagliptin on glycaemic control in patients with type 2 diabetes and chronic kidney disease (DELIGHT): a randomised, double-blind, placebo-controlled trial. Lancet Diabetes Endocrinol 2019;7(6):429–41.

65. Kohler S, Zeller C, Iliev H, et al. Safety and tolerability of empagliflozin in patients with type 2 diabetes: pooled analysis of phase I-III clinical trials. Adv Ther 2017;34(7):1707–26.

66. Yabe D, Yasui A, Ji L, et al. Safety and tolerability of empagliflozin in East Asian patients with type 2 diabetes: pooled analysis of phase I-III clinical trials. J Diabetes Investig 2019;10(2):418–28.

67. Kashiwagi A, Shestakova MV, Ito Y, et al. Safety of ipragliflozin in patients with type 2 diabetes mellitus: pooled Analysis of Phase II/III/IV Clinical Trials. Diabetes Ther 2019;10(6):2201–17.

68. Dorsey-Treviño EG, González-González JG, Alvarez-Villalobos N, et al. Sodium-glucose cotransporter 2 (SGLT-2) inhibitors and microvascular outcomes in patients with type 2 diabetes: systematic review and meta-analysis. J Endocrinol Invest 2020;43(3):289–304.

69. Qiu M, Ding LL, Zhang M, et al. Safety of four SGLT2 inhibitors in three chronic diseases: a meta-analysis of large randomized trials of SGLT2 inhibitors. Diab Vasc Dis Res 2021;18(2). 14791641211011016.

70. McGuire DK, Shih WJ, Cosentino F, et al. Association of SGLT2 inhibitors with cardiovascular and kidney outcomes in patients with type 2 diabetes: a meta-analysis. JAMA Cardiol 2021;6(2):148–58.

71. Udell JA, Yuan Z, Rush T, et al. Cardiovascular outcomes and risks after initiation of a sodium glucose co-transporter 2 inhibitor: results from the easel population-based cohort study. Circulation 2018;137(14):1450–9.

72. Adimadhyam S, Lee TA, Calip GS, et al. Risk of amputations associated with SGLT2 inhibitors compared to DPP-4 inhibitors: A propensity-matched cohort study. Diabetes Obes Metab 2018;20(12):2792–9.

73. Yu OHY, Dell'Aniello S, Shah BR, et al. Sodium-glucose cotransporter 2 inhibitors and the risk of below-knee amputation: a multicenter observational study. Diabetes care 2020;43(10):2444–52.

74. Udell JA, Yuan Z, Ryan P, et al. Cardiovascular outcomes and mortality after initiation of canagliflozin: analyses from the EASEL study. Endocrinol Diabetes Metab 2020;3(1):e00096.

75. Werkman NCC, Nielen JTH, van den Bergh JPW, et al. Use of sodium-glucose co-transporter-2-inhibitors (SGLT2-Is) and risk of lower limb amputation. Curr Drug Saf 2021;16(1):62–72.

Sodium-glucose Cotransporter 2 Inhibitors and Nonalcoholic Fatty Liver Disease

Husam M. Salah, MD[a], Marat Fudim, MD, MHS[b,c],*

KEYWORDS

- SGLT2 inhibitors • Nonalcoholic fatty liver disease • NAFLD • Mechanisms • Pathophysiology

KEY POINTS

- NAFLD is being more recognized as a systematic and cardiovascular disease and not only a hepatic disease with a complex pathophysiology and no effective pharmacotherapy to date.
- Preclinical and clinical studies suggest a promising role for SGLT2 inhibitors in NAFLD.
- This review proposes the following mechanisms as drivers for SGLT2 inhibitor effects in NAFLD: increasing insulin sensitivity, decreasing fat accumulation in the liver and liptotixicty, decreasing oxidative stress and ER stress, improving autophagy, and inhibiting apoptosis.
- Large-scale randomized controlled trials are needed to establish the efficacy of SGLT2 inhibitors in patients with NAFLD.

INTRODUCTION

Nonalcoholic fatty liver disease (NAFLD) is the most common chronic liver disease worldwide and is a leading cause of morbidity and mortality with a global prevalence of 25%.[1] NAFLD includes a spectrum of liver conditions that range from simple hepatic steatosis (ie, intrahepatic fat ≥5% of liver weight) to nonalcoholic steatohepatitis (NASH), which is defined histologically as hepatic steatosis and necroinflammation with or without hepatic fibrosis[2]; progression of NASH can lead to cirrhosis (**Fig. 1**).[2]

NAFLD is becoming more recognized as not only a hepatic disorder but also a cardiovascular and systemic disorder that is closely related to cardiovascular diseases, including coronary artery disease and incident heart failure.[3–5] Although the pathophysiological mechanisms underlying NAFLD are complex and multifactorial, insulin resistance, intrahepatic fat accumulation, lipotoxicity, mitochondrial dysfunction, oxidative stress, endoplasmic reticulum (ER) stress, abnormal autophagy, altered gut flora, and apoptosis seem to be key processes involved in the development and progression of different stages of NAFLD.[6–8] Despite that several pharmacologic therapies have been investigated as a potential treatment for NAFLD (eg, metformin, thiazolidinediones, the antioxidant vitamin E) with various others under investigation (eg, caspase inhibitors and farnesoid X receptor agonists), effective pharmacotherapy for NAFLD remains lacking.[9]

In addition to the well-established association between NAFLD and atherosclerotic cardiovascular disease, an accumulating body of evidence suggests as an association between NAFLD and heart failure.[3,4] A recent population-based

Financial support: none.
[a] Department of Medicine, University of Arkansas for Medical Sciences, Little Rock, AR, USA; [b] Division of Cardiology, Department of Medicine, Duke University, Durham, NC, USA; [c] Duke Clinical Research Institute, Durham, NC, USA
* Corresponding author. Division of Cardiology, Duke University School of Medicine, Duke Clinical Research Institute, MHS, 2301 Erwin Road, Durham, NC, 27705.
E-mail address: marat.fudim@gmail.com

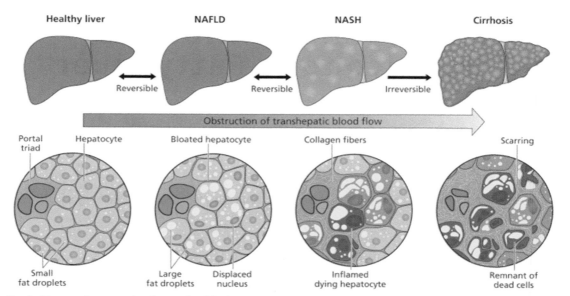

Fig. 1. Stages of progression from a healthy liver to cirrhosis due to nonalcoholic fatty liver disease. (*From* Salah HM, Pandey A, Soloveva A, Abdelmalek MF, Diehl AM, Moylan CA, Wegermann K, Rao VN, Hernandez AF, Tedford RJ, Parikh KS, Mentz RJ, McGarrah RW, Fudim M. Relationship of Nonalcoholic Fatty Liver Disease and Heart Failure With Preserved Ejection Fraction. JACC Basic Transl Sci. 2021 Nov 22;6(11):918-932.)

analysis showed that patients with NAFLD are at 24% increased risk of new-onset heart failure after adjustment for several clinical and demographic factors[4]; when analyzed based on heart failure phenotype, NAFLD had a stronger association with heart failure with preserved ejection fraction (HFpEF) compared with heart failure with reduced ejection fraction (HFrEF),[4] which suggests that NAFLD may be a precursor and driver for some HFpEF phenotypes (**Fig. 2**). NAFLD and heart failure (specifically HFpEF) share several pathophysiological mechanisms and features, such as inflammation, endothelial dysfunction, and excess epicardial adipose tissue, which may underlie the association between these two entities.[3]

Sodium-glucose cotransporter 2 (SGLT2) inhibitors have established cardiovascular benefits in patients with and without diabetes, patients with acute and chronic heart failure across a wide spectrum of left ventricular ejection fraction, and patients with and without atherosclerotic cardiovascular disease (**Fig. 3**).[10–13] Given the robust evidence establishing the cardiovascular protective effects of SGLT2 inhibitors in patients with diseases that share similar pathophysiological mechanisms as NAFLD and the lack of an effective pharmacotherapy for NAFLD,[11,12] a growing interest in investigating the role of SGLT2 inhibitors in NAFLD has been undertaken with promising signals of favorable effects in preclinical and clinical studies. In this review, we summarize the current evidence of the effect of SGLT2 inhibitors on

NAFLD and propose several mechanisms that may explain their favorable effects.

DO SODIUM-GLUCOSE COTRANSPORTER 2 INHIBITORS ALSO WORK IN NONALCOHOLIC FATTY LIVER DISEASE?
Evidence from Preclinical Studies

Most of the evidence on the effectiveness of SGLT2 inhibitors in the treatment of NAFLD and the potential mechanisms of action that underly this effect are derived from preclinical models. Herein, we summarize the available evidence from various preclinical models.

Several preclinical models demonstrated the effects of SGLT2 inhibitors on hepatic lipid metabolism in NAFLD. In a mice model, oleic acid (OA) significantly increased intracellular lipid accumulation and triglycerides content[14]; a 4-week treatment with dapagliflozin remarkably decreased OA-induced lipid accumulation and triglycerides content.[14] On the molecular level, dapagliflozin resulted in a decrease in the expression of critical lipogenic transcription factors (ie, sterol regulatory element-binding protein 1 (SREBP-1c), peroxisome proliferator-activated receptor alpha (PPARα)) and their downstream enzymes.[14] Dapagliflozin also activated adenosine monophosphate-activated protein kinase (AMPK) phosphorylation but inhibited mammalian target of rapamycin (mTOR) phosphorylation,[14] both of which are key regulators of energy metabolism

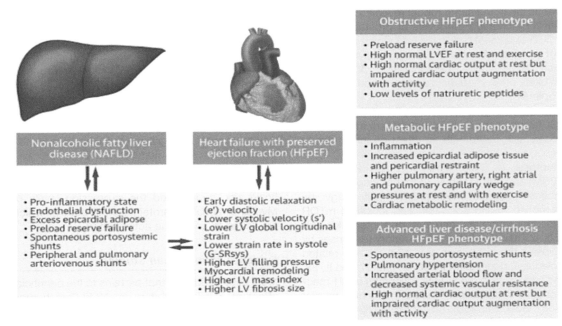

Fig. 2. The association between nonalcoholic fatty liver disease and heart failure with preserved ejection fraction. LV, left ventricle; LVEF left ventricular ejection fraction. (*From* Salah HM, Pandey A, Soloveva A, Abdelmalek MF, Diehl AM, Moylan CA, Wegermann K, Rao VN, Hernandez AF, Tedford RJ, Parikh KS, Mentz RJ, McGarrah RW, Fudim M. Relationship of Nonalcoholic Fatty Liver Disease and Heart Failure With Preserved Ejection Fraction. JACC Basic Transl Sci. 2021 Nov 22;6(11):918-932.)

and a target for NAFLD.[14] The findings in this model suggest that dapagliflozin significantly ameliorates hepatic steatosis through its effect on the AMPK/mTOR pathway. In a nonobese prediabetic rat model, an 8-week treatment with empagliflozin significantly reduced lipotoxic diacylglycerols and neutral triacylglycerols in the liver along with changes in mRNA expression of lipogenic enzymes, alterations in cytochrome P450 proteins, and a decrease in the circulating levels of fetuin-A[15]; these changes were associated with improvement in hepatic lipid metabolism and attenuation of insulin resistance in the liver as well as peripheral tissues. This model suggests that empagliflozin may play a role in alleviating NAFLD manifestations in the early phase of the disease.[15] In obese diabetic mice, canagliflozin attenuated hepatic fat deposition in the absence of a reduction in body or fat weight, which suggests that the reduction in hepatic fat accumulation associated with canagliflozin is independent of body and fat weight.[16] Lipidomics analysis of

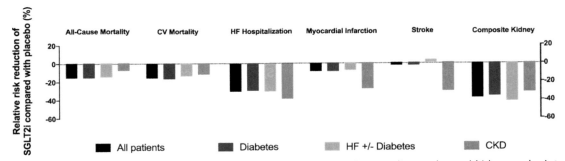

Fig. 3. The effect of sodium-glucose cotransporter 2 inhibitors on various cardiovascular and kidney endpoints compared with placebo. CKD, chronic kidney disease; CV, cardiovascular; HF, heart failure; SGLT2i, sodium-glucose cotransporter 2 inhibitor. (*From* Salah HM, Al'Aref SJ, Khan MS, Al-Hawwas M, Vallurupalli S, Mehta JL, Mounsey JP, Greene SJ, McGuire DK, Lopes RD, Fudim M. Effect of sodium-glucose cotransporter 2 inhibitors on cardiovascular and kidney outcomes-Systematic review and meta-analysis of randomized placebo-controlled trials. Am Heart J. 2021 Feb;232:10-22.)

liver tissue in the same model revealed that cana-gliflozin increased the levels of prostaglandin E2 (PGE2) and resolvin E3, both of which are important lipid mediators.[16] In vitro analysis of the mice hepatocytes demonstrated that PGE2 inhibited the hepatic accumulation of lipid droplets.[16]

The following models showed that the effect of SGLT2 inhibitors on lipid metabolism in NAFLD is closely associated with an effect on inflammatory response, oxidative stress, autophagy, and apoptosis. A mice model of type 2 diabetes (T2DM) and NAFLD showed that empagliflozin can enhance hepatic macrophages autophagy by promoting AMPK activation and inhibiting mTOR phosphorylation and can suppress interleukin (IL)-17/IL-23 axis-mediated inflammatory responses by inhibiting the expression of IL-17/IL-23 axis-related molecules, decreasing the level of IL-17 and IL-23, and suppressing the hepatic infiltration of M1 macrophages and T-helper 17 cells.[17] In a high-fat diet mice model, empagliflozin decreased NAFLD activity score compared with placebo[18]; it also decreased the expression of lipogenic enzymes and ER stress molecules as well as inflammatory molecules.[18] Empagliflozin also activated autophagy via promoting AMPK phosphorylation, decreasing mTOR expression, and increasing microtubule-associated protein 1 light chain 3B (LC3B) expression, and reduced liver cell apoptosis via increasing the Bcl2/Bax ratio and inhibiting CASPASE-8 cleavage.[18] In Zucker diabetic fatty rats, dapagliflozin reduced hepatic lipid accumulation via upregulating genes related to fatty acid oxidation (eg, lipid β-oxidation enzyme acyl-CoA oxidase 1) and downregulating the expression of hepatic lipogenic genes (eg, acetyl-CoA carboxylase 1)[19]; dapagliflozin also increased the expression of autophagy-related markers (ie, LC3B and Beclin1). In a mice model, canagliflozin resulted in a dose-dependent attenuation of hepatic oxidative stress and upregulation of the antioxidant enzymes activity and the total antioxidant capacity.[20]

The beneficial effects of SGLT2 inhibitors extend to the advanced stages of steatosis as evidenced by a nondiabetic, biopsy-confirmed mice model of advanced NASH, in which empagliflozin improved the NAFLD activity score[21]; the improvement in the NAFLD activity score was mainly driven by lower scores in liver lobular inflammation rather than in liver steatosis.[21] Empagliflozin decreased the hepatic levels of the proinflammatory lactosylceramides and increased the levels of the anti-inflammatory polyunsaturated triglycerides.[21] In another study in mice with T2DM and NASH, ipragliflozin significantly improved hepatic steatosis and fibrosis and attenuated inflammation

and oxidative stress in the liver.[22] These results suggest that in advanced stages on hepatic steatosis, the beneficial effects of SGLT2 inhibitors could be mainly driven by attenuating inflammation, which may subsequently inhibit the progression to liver fibrosis.

SGLT2 inhibitors may also suppress the development of NASH-associated hepatocellular carcinoma. In a mouse model of human NASH, a 1-year treatment with canagliflozin resulted in a significant reduction in the number of liver tumors with a trend toward smaller tumor sizes in the canagliflozin groups compared with placebo.[23] Canagliflozin also suppressed the expression levels of Myc and alpha fetoprotein genes, both of which are linked to oncogene activation.[23]

Evidence from Human Studies

Most of the evidence that pertains to the beneficial effect of SGLT2 inhibitors on NAFLD in human studies is derived from studies on patients with T2DM.

SGLT2 inhibitors exert a beneficial effect related to NAFLD in all stages, including the pre-NAFLD stage as demonstrated by a large UK cohort study showing that the use of SGLT2 inhibitors is associated with a 22% lower hazards of incident NAFLD among patients with T2DM.[24]

In the randomized controlled E-LIFE trial, which randomized 50 patients with T2DM and NAFLD to receive either empagliflozin and standard treatment of T2DM or standard treatment of T2DM without empagliflozin for 20 weeks, there was a significant reduction in liver fat (as assessed by magnetic resonance imaging [MRI]-proton density fat fraction [PDFF]) in the empagliflozin group compared with baseline (16.2% to 11.3%; $P < .0001$) but no significant change was seen in the control group (16.4% to 15.5%; $P = .057$).[25] In another randomized controlled trial of 32 patients with T2DM and NAFLD who were randomized to either luseogliflozin or metformin, luseogliflozin resulted in a greater favorable change in the liver-to-spleen attenuation ratio (L/S) obtained by computed tomography[26]; L/S is a validated approach in diagnosing the presence of liver fat with an L/S < 1.0 diagnosing the presence of liver fat.[27] In a meta-analysis of randomized controlled trials evaluating the effectiveness of various antidiabetic agents for the treatment of NAFLD in patients with type 2 diabetes, SGLT2 inhibitors resulted in a significant reduction in steatosis compared with standard of care with a mean difference of −2.6%.[28]

The favorable effects of SGLT2 inhibitors on NAFLD were shown using different fibrosis indices and assessment techniques. In patients with NAFLD and T2DM, empagliflozin resulted in a significant decrease in controlled attenuation parameter (CAP; 282.07 ± 47.29 dB/m vs 263.07 ± 49.93 dB/m) and liver stiffness (5.89 ± 4.23 kPa vs 5.04 ± 1.49 kPa) using FibroScan at 6 months.[29] In a propensity score-matched analysis of 56 patients with NAFLD and T2DM, SGLT2 inhibitors were associated with a significant improvement in fibrosis-4 (FIB-4) index, a noninvasive scoring system for liver fibrosis, and reduction in the liver stiffness measurement (LSM) and CAP as assessed through transient elastography using FibroScan.[30] In a 6-month prospective single-arm study that included six patients with T2DM and NAFLD, canagliflozin resulted in a significant reduction in hepatic PDFF as assessed by MRI after 6 months of treatment[31]; PDFF can reliably provide estimation and quantification of the liver fat content.[32] In another retrospective analysis of 637 patients with T2DM who were switched from metformin to either dipeptidyl-peptidase-4 (DPP-4) inhibitors, GLP-1 receptor agonists, or SGLT2 inhibitors, GLP-1 receptor agonists and SGLT2 inhibitors significantly reduced FIB-4 score and fatty liver index (compared with both controls and DPP-4 inhibitors) with persistent effect after adjustment for propensity score.[33] In patients with T2DM, empagliflozin significantly reduced liver fat content with no effect on epicardial, myocardial or pancreatic fat content as assessed by MRI with magnetic resonance spectroscopy (MRS)[34]; these findings suggest possible tissue-specific mobilization of fat stores exerted by SGLT2 inhibitors and support the accumulating evidence of the direct effect of SGLT2 inhibitors on the hepatic lipid and fat metabolism.

Empagliflozin use in patients with T2DM and NAFLD can result in a significant decrease in liver enzymes (serum alanine aminotransferase [ALT], aspartate aminotransferase [AST], and gamma-glutamyl transferase [GGT]) among these patients.[29] In a Korean population study including patients with T2DM-associated NAFLD on metformin therapy who required a stepwise addition of other oral antidiabetic agents, the use of SGLT2 inhibitors (compared with other oral antidiabetic agents) was associated with a greater decrease in ALT levels, and the use of SGLT2 inhibitors was an independent factor of ALT improvement in a multivariate logistic regression model.[35]

The effects of SGLT2 inhibitors on NAFLD appear to extend to include the more severe form of NAFLD (ie, NASH); however, the evidence is scant in NASH. In a prospective study including 10 patients with biopsy-confirmed NASH (hepatic fibrosis stages 1–3) and T2DM, in which treatment with canagliflozin for 12 weeks resulted in significant improvements in FIB-4 index and FM-fibro index, both of which are validated indices for liver fibrosis.[36]

There is also limited evidence regarding the efficacy of SGLT2 inhibitors in patients with NAFLD but no T2DM. In one study including 10 overweight, insulin-resistant patients without T2DM, a 12-week treatment with dapagliflozin did not result in a reduction in hepatic steatosis (assessed using MRS) with no change in the global measures of lipid oxidation.[37] Although more studies are needed in this population before drawing a conclusion, the absence of an effect for dapagliflozin on hepatic steatosis along with no effect on lipid oxidation in patients with NAFLD but no T2DM (as opposed to those with NAFLD and T2DM) may suggest that the favorable effects of SGLT2 inhibitors on NAFLD may largely be driven by their ability to counteract many of the underlying hepatic pathophysiological processes that are mainly mediated by hyperglycemia and insulin resistance.

The beneficial effects of SGLT2 inhibitors on NAFLD were also demonstrated histopathologically. In a retrospective small study of seven patients with NAFLD and T2DM who were treated with canagliflozin and in whom liver biopsies were obtained at the three different points (ie, pretreatment, 24 weeks, and ≥1 year after the initiation of canagliflozin),[38] although the seven patients had worsening of body mass index and waist circumference over the study period, canagliflozin was associated with long-term liver histopathological improvement (ie, steatosis, lobular inflammation, ballooning, and fibrosis) at the third biopsy in six of seven patients.[38] These histopathological changes were also seen in patients with NASH; in a single-arm, open-label study in nine patients with biopsy-proven NASH and T2DM, a 24-week of empagliflozin resulted in a significant reduction in volumetric liver fat fraction, steatosis, ballooning, and fibrosis on liver biopsy at the end of treatment.[39]

PROPOSED MECHANISMS FOR THE FAVORABLE EFFECTS OF SGLT2 IN NONALCOHOLIC FATTY LIVER DISEASE

The exact mechanisms by which SGLT2 inhibitors exert their beneficial effects on NAFLD are not well understood. In this section, we propose the following mechanisms based on our understanding of NAFLD pathogenesis and the current available evidence from preclinical models that support possible mechanisms. The pathogenesis of NAFLD is multifactorial with diverse parallel processes that involve insulin resistance, fat accumulation in the liver (especially triglycerides), increased lipotoxicity, mitochondrial dysfunction, oxidative stress, ER stress, abnormal autophagy, altered gut flora, activation of hepatic stellate cells, and apoptosis (**Fig. 4**).[6–8]

Evidence from preclinical models suggests that SGLT2 inhibitors can counteract NAFLD by increasing insulin sensitivity, decreasing fat accumulation in the liver, decreasing liptotixicty, oxidative stress, and ER stress, improving autophagy, and inhibiting apoptosis. SGLT2 inhibitors likely achieve these endpoints through the following pathways:

Improving Insulin Sensitivity

Insulin resistance is one of the mainstay mechanisms of NAFLD pathogenesis and is involved in different other pathogenic mechanisms of NAFLD, such as inflammation, oxidative stress, and hepatic fat accumulation. Although preclinical models have demonstrated that SGLT2 inhibitors exert an insulin-sensitizing effect,[40,41] human studies are nonconclusive with possible tissue-specific effects.[42,43] Current evidence signals for a possible effect of SGLT2 inhibitors on improving insulin resistance and β-cell function by promoting the expression of various β-cell-related factors, polarizing M2 macrophages and restoring the balance of adipocyte-derived hormones (ie, leptin, fibroblast growth factor 21, and adiponectin).[44]

Increasing Glucagon/Insulin Ratio

SGLT-2 is expressed in the pancreatic α-cells, which secrete glucagon.[45] SGLT2 inhibitors act as alpha cell secretagogue promoting glucagon secretion with subsequent suppression in insulin secretion.[45] The increase in glucagon/insulin ratio can subsequently induce a transition in metabolism from carbohydrate to lipid metabolism and an increase in energy expenditure[46], due to this transition, fatty acid oxidation is activated along with a reduction in hepatic triglycerides.[47] As fat accumulation in the liver (specifically triglycerides) is a key mechanism in the development and progression of NAFLD, the increase in glucagon/insulin ratio along with fatty acid oxidation and reduction in hepatic triglycerides would counteract this key pathogenic mechanism.

Regulating AMPK/mTOR Pathway

As discussed in the preclinical studies, several preclinical studies showed that SGLT2 inhibitors can activate AMPK phosphorylation and inhibit mTOR phosphorylation and expression.[14,17–19] Both AMPK and mTOR are important energy sensors and regulators of metabolic homeostasis[48–50]; mTOR is also involved in de novo lipid synthesis in the liver.[49] There is a growing body of evidence suggesting that AMPK activity is suppressed in metabolic disorders (eg, NAFLD) and that its activation improves lipid dysregulation, inflammation, hepatic injury, and fibrosis in NAFLD,[48] whereas chronic activation of mTOR is prevalent in metabolic disorders.[50] In addition, AMPK promotes autophagy,[51] although mTOR is a negative regulator of autophagy.[52] The activation of AMPK and suppression of the expression and activity of mTOR would restore the abnormal autophagy function in NAFLD. This was evidenced by enhancement in autophagy as a consequence of AMPK activation and mTOR inhibition following SGLT2 inhibitors use in animal studies.[17–19]

Browning of White Adipose Tissue

Low brown adipose tissue activity is associated with increased fat accumulation in the human liver,[53] and patients with NAFLD have lower brown

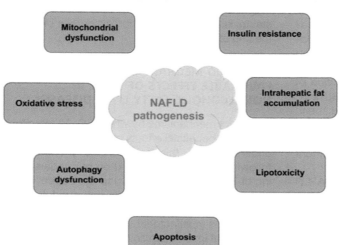

Fig. 4. Pathogenesis of nonalcohol fatty liver disease. NAFLD, nonalcohol fatty liver disease.

adipose tissue activity compared with controls.[53] Although the effect of SGLT2 inhibitors on brown adipose tissue activity has not been directly studied in human, in an obese mice model, a 4-week treatment with dapagliflozin resulted in enhancement in fat utilization and browning of white adipose tissue without significant disturbance in plasma glycolipid level or weight gain.[54] This suggests that SGLT2 inhibitors may counteract hepatic fat accumulation by the browning of white adipose tissue.

Attenuating Hepatic Inflammation

Inflammation is a key factor in the development and progress of NAFLD.[55] Although the inflammatory mediators in NAFLD are likely derived from multifactorial processes, adipocytokine synthesis, increased lipid storage, and lipogenesis are central to these processes.[55] As discussed before, SGLT2 inhibitors can decrease hepatic lipid storage, inhibit de novo lipid synthesis, and increase lipid metabolism and fatty acid oxidation. These processes cumulatively attenuate hepatic inflammation as evidenced by preclinical models demonstrating suppression of the IL-17/IL-23 axis-mediated inflammatory responses, decrease hepatic infiltration of M1 macrophages and T helper 17 cells, reduction in the levels of the pro-inflammatory lactosylceramides, increase in the levels of the anti-inflammatory polyunsaturated triglycerides, and attenuation of liver lobular inflammation associated with SGLT2 inhibitors use.[17,18,21,22]

Decreasing Oxidative Stress

Oxidative stress is another key factor in NAFLD pathogenesis and stems from multiple pathophysiological mechanisms, mainly mitochondrial dysfunction, ER stress, inflammation, iron metabolism derangements, insulin resistance, and endothelial dysfunction.[56] Evidence suggests that SGLT2 inhibitors can counteract at least some of these mechanisms. In addition to its role in improving insulin sensitivity and attenuating inflammation and thus reducing oxidative stress; a growing body of evidence suggests that SGLT2 inhibitors can improve mitochondrial dysfunction, optimize mitochondrial energy utilization, improve mitochondrial energetics and mitochondrial oxidative defense.[56,57] Also, the previously discussed preclinical models showed that SGLT2 inhibitors can upregulate antioxidant enzymes and decrease the expression of ER stress molecules.[18,20]

Inhibiting Apoptosis

Hepatocyte apoptosis is closely associated with NAFLD and NASH development and progression.[58] Apoptotic hepatocytes stimulate an immune response and activate hepatic stellate cells with subsequent production and secretion of inflammasomes and cytokines, which results in fibrosis.[58] SGLT2 inhibitors can inhibit apoptosis by increasing the Bcl2/Bax ratio and inhibiting CASPASE-8 cleavage. Bcl2/Bax ratio determines cell susceptibility to apoptosis with higher levels denoting a lower susceptibility to apoptosis,[59] whereas activation of CASPASE-8 propagates the apoptotic signal and activates downstream key regulators of apoptosis.[60]

FUTURE DIRECTIONS

There are several gaps in the literature regarding the use of SGLT2 inhibitors in NAFLD. Although the current evidence suggests a potential role for SGLT2 inhibitors in the treatment of NAFLD, the efficacy and safety of SGLT2 inhibitors in this setting have not been evaluated yet in large-scale randomized controlled trials. Further, the available evidence in humans is mostly driven from studies in patients with concurrent T2DM. Although NAFLD and T2DM co-exist very commonly and share several pathophysiological mechanisms,[61] studies aiming at elucidating the effects of SGLT2 inhibitors in patients with NAFLD without T2DM and uncovering the mechanisms of these effects outside the context of T2DM are needed. The NCT04642261 is an ongoing randomized trial that aims to investigate the effect of empagliflozin on liver fat in patients without T2DM. NAFLD has been proposed as a potential driver of de novo heart failure.[3,4] As the current evidence suggests that SGLT2 inhibitors can decrease the risk of incident heart failure,[62] it is possible that the use of SGLT2 inhibitors in patients with NAFLD without concurrent heart failure may be associated with a more pronounced reduction in the risk of incidence heart failure from the baseline risk compared with those without NAFLD; studies investigating this hypothesis are needed.

SUMMARY

NAFLD is not only a hepatic disorder but also a systemic and cardiovascular disease with a growing global burden and no effective pharmacotherapy to date. The lack of an effective pharmacotherapy is, in part, because of complex and multifactorial pathophysiological mechanisms that drive NAFLD. These mechanisms involve insulin resistance, intrahepatic fat accumulation, lipotoxicity, mitochondrial dysfunction, oxidative stress, ER stress, abnormal autophagy, altered gut flora, and apoptosis. Current evidence suggests that SGLT2 inhibitors may be a promising

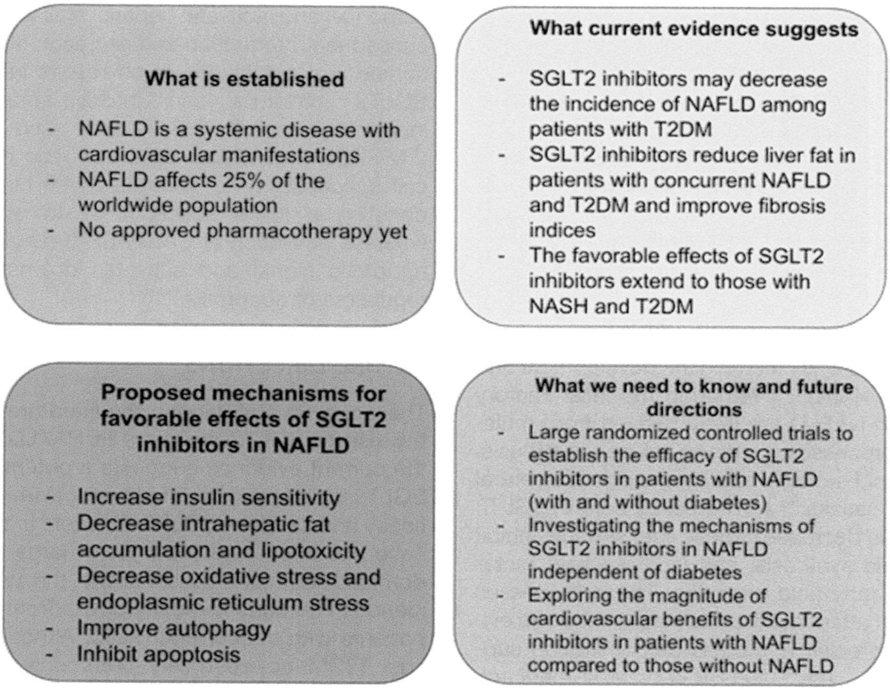

What is established

- NAFLD is a systemic disease with cardiovascular manifestations
- NAFLD affects 25% of the worldwide population
- No approved pharmacotherapy yet

What current evidence suggests

- SGLT2 inhibitors may decrease the incidence of NAFLD among patients with T2DM
- SGLT2 inhibitors reduce liver fat in patients with concurrent NAFLD and T2DM and improve fibrosis indices
- The favorable effects of SGLT2 inhibitors extend to those with NASH and T2DM

Proposed mechanisms for favorable effects of SGLT2 inhibitors in NAFLD

- Increase insulin sensitivity
- Decrease intrahepatic fat accumulation and lipotoxicity
- Decrease oxidative stress and endoplasmic reticulum stress
- Improve autophagy
- Inhibit apoptosis

What we need to know and future directions

- Large randomized controlled trials to establish the efficacy of SGLT2 inhibitors in patients with NAFLD (with and without diabetes)
- Investigating the mechanisms of SGLT2 inhibitors in NAFLD independent of diabetes
- Exploring the magnitude of cardiovascular benefits of SGLT2 inhibitors in patients with NAFLD compared to those without NAFLD

Fig. 5. A center figure summarizing the key points of this review.

treatment for NAFLD, potentially via their ability to increase insulin sensitivity, decrease fat accumulation in the liver and lipotoxicity, decrease oxidative stress and ER stress, improve autophagy, and inhibit apoptosis (**Fig. 5**).

CLINICS CARE POINTS

- NAFLD should be recognized as a systemic disease with cardiovascular manifestations.
- SGLT2 inhibitors should be considered in patients with NAFLD and a comorbidity with an approved indication (eg, T2DM, HFrEF).
- The efficacy of SGLT2 inhibitors in patients with NAFLD but no T2DM is uncertain.

DISCLOSURE

M. Fudim was supported by NHLBI K23HL151744 from the National Heart, Lung, and Blood Institute (NHLBI), the American Heart Association grant No 20IPA35310955, Mario Family Award, Duke Chair's Award, Translating Duke Health Award, Bayer, and BTG Specialty Pharmaceuticals. He receives consulting fees from AstraZeneca, AxonTherapies, CVRx, Daxor, Edwards LifeSciences, Galvani, NXT Biomedical, Zoll, and Viscardia. H.M. Salah declares no disclosures.

REFERENCES

1. Younossi ZM, Koenig AB, Abdelatif D, et al. Global epidemiology of nonalcoholic fatty liver disease-Meta-analytic assessment of prevalence, incidence, and outcomes. Hepatology 2016;64(1):73–84.
2. Diehl AM, Day C. Cause, Pathogenesis, and Treatment of Nonalcoholic Steatohepatitis. N Engl J Med 2017;377(21):2063–72.
3. Salah HM, Pandey A, Soloveva A, et al. Relationship of nonalcoholic fatty liver disease and heart failure with preserved ejection fraction. JACC: Basic Translational Sci 2021;6(11):918–32.
4. Fudim M, Zhong L, Patel KV, et al. Nonalcoholic Fatty Liver Disease and Risk of Heart Failure Among Medicare Beneficiaries. J Am Heart Assoc 2021; 10(22):e021654.
5. Tana C, Ballestri S, Ricci F, et al. Cardiovascular Risk in Non-Alcoholic Fatty Liver Disease: Mechanisms and Therapeutic Implications. Int J Environ Res Public Health 2019;16(17):3104.
6. Tessari P, Coracina A, Cosma A, et al. Hepatic lipid metabolism and non-alcoholic fatty liver disease. Nutr Metab Cardiovasc Dis 2009;19(4):291–302.
7. Buzzetti E, Pinzani M, Tsochatzis EA. The multiple-hit pathogenesis of non-alcoholic fatty liver disease (NAFLD). Metabolism 2016;65(8):1038–48.
8. Yan S, Huda N, Khambu B, et al. Relevance of autophagy to fatty liver diseases and potential therapeutic applications. Amino Acids 2017; 49(12):1965–79.

9. Attia SL, Softic S, Mouzaki M. Evolving Role for Pharmacotherapy in NAFLD/NASH. Clin Transl Sci 2021; 14(1):11–9.

10. Zelniker TA, Wiviott SD, Raz I, et al. SGLT2 inhibitors for primary and secondary prevention of cardiovascular and renal outcomes in type 2 diabetes: a systematic review and meta-analysis of cardiovascular outcome trials. Lancet 2019;393(10166):31–9.

11. Salah HM, Al'Aref SJ, Khan MS, et al. Effect of sodium-glucose cotransporter 2 inhibitors on cardiovascular and kidney outcomes—Systematic review and meta-analysis of randomized placebo-controlled trials. Am Heart J 2021;232:10–22.

12. Salah HM, Al'Aref SJ, Khan MS, et al. Effects of sodium-glucose cotransporter 1 and 2 inhibitors on cardiovascular and kidney outcomes in type 2 diabetes: A meta-analysis update. Am Heart J 2021; 233:86–91.

13. Salah HM, Al'Aref SJ, Khan MS, et al. Efficacy and safety of sodium-glucose cotransporter 2 inhibitors initiation in patients with acute heart failure, with and without type 2 diabetes: a systematic review and meta-analysis. Cardiovasc Diabetol 2022; 21(1):20.

14. Luo J, Sun P, Wang Y, et al. Dapagliflozin attenuates steatosis in livers of high-fat diet-induced mice and oleic acid-treated L02 cells via regulating AMPK/mTOR pathway. Eur J Pharmacol 2021;907:174304.

15. Hüttl M, Markova I, Miklankova D, et al. In a Prediabetic Model, Empagliflozin Improves Hepatic Lipid Metabolism Independently of Obesity and before Onset of Hyperglycemia. Int J Mol Sci 2021;22(21).

16. Yoshino K, Hosooka T, Shinohara M, et al. Canagliflozin ameliorates hepatic fat deposition in obese diabetic mice: Role of prostaglandin E(2). Biochem Biophys Res Commun 2021;557:62–8.

17. Meng Z, Liu X, Li T, et al. The SGLT2 inhibitor empagliflozin negatively regulates IL-17/IL-23 axis-mediated inflammatory responses in T2DM with NAFLD via the AMPK/mTOR/autophagy pathway. Int Immunopharmacol 2021;94:107492.

18. Nasiri-Ansari N, Nikolopoulou C, Papoutsi K, et al. Empagliflozin Attenuates Non-Alcoholic Fatty Liver Disease (NAFLD) in High Fat Diet Fed ApoE((-/-)) Mice by Activating Autophagy and Reducing ER Stress and Apoptosis. Int J Mol Sci 2021;22(2).

19. Li L, Li Q, Huang W, et al. Dapagliflozin Alleviates Hepatic Steatosis by Restoring Autophagy via the AMPK-mTOR Pathway. Front Pharmacol 2021;12: 589273.

20. Kabil SL, Mahmoud NM. Canagliflozin protects against non-alcoholic steatohepatitis in type-2 diabetic rats through zinc alpha-2 glycoprotein upregulation. Eur J Pharmacol 2018;828:135–45.

21. Perakakis N, Chrysafi P, Feigh M, et al. Empagliflozin Improves Metabolic and Hepatic Outcomes in a Non-Diabetic Obese Biopsy-Proven Mouse Model of Advanced NASH. Int J Mol Sci 2021;22(12):6332.

22. Tahara A, Takasu T. Therapeutic Effects of SGLT2 Inhibitor Ipragliflozin and Metformin on NASH in Type 2 Diabetic Mice. Endocr Res 2020;45(2):147–61.

23. Shiba K, Tsuchiya K, Komiya C, et al. Canagliflozin, an SGLT2 inhibitor, attenuates the development of hepatocellular carcinoma in a mouse model of human NASH. Sci Rep 2018;8(1):2362.

24. Pradhan R, Yin H, Yu O, et al. Glucagon-Like Peptide 1 Receptor Agonists and Sodium–Glucose Cotransporter 2 Inhibitors and Risk of Nonalcoholic Fatty Liver Disease Among Patients With Type 2 Diabetes. Diabetes Care 2022;45(4):819–29.

25. Kuchay MS, Krishan S, Mishra SK, et al. Effect of Empagliflozin on Liver Fat in Patients With Type 2 Diabetes and Nonalcoholic Fatty Liver Disease: A Randomized Controlled Trial (E-LIFT Trial). Diabetes Care 2018;41(8):1801–8.

26. Shibuya T, Fushimi N, Kawai M, et al. Luseogliflozin improves liver fat deposition compared to metformin in type 2 diabetes patients with non-alcoholic fatty liver disease: A prospective randomized controlled pilot study. Diabetes Obes Metab 2018;20(2): 438–42.

27. Zeb I, Li D, Nasir K, et al. Computed tomography scans in the evaluation of fatty liver disease in a population based study: the multi-ethnic study of atherosclerosis. Acad Radiol 2012;19(7):811–8.

28. Ng CH, Lin SY, Chin YH, et al. Antidiabetic Medications for Type 2 Diabetics with Nonalcoholic Fatty Liver Disease: Evidence From a Network Meta-Analysis of Randomized Controlled Trials. Endocr Pract 2022;28(2):223–30.

29. Pokharel A, Kc S, Thapa P, et al. The Effect of Empagliflozin on Liver Fat in Type 2 Diabetes Mellitus Patients With Non-Alcoholic Fatty Liver Disease. Cureus 2021;13(7):e16687.

30. Arai T, Atsukawa M, Tsubota A, et al. Effect of sodium-glucose cotransporter 2 inhibitor in patients with non-alcoholic fatty liver disease and type 2 diabetes mellitus: a propensity score-matched analysis of real-world data. Ther Adv Endocrinol Metab 2021; 12. 20420188211000243.

31. Nishimiya N, Tajima K, Imajo K, et al. Effects of Canagliflozin on Hepatic Steatosis, Visceral Fat and Skeletal Muscle among Patients with Type 2 Diabetes and Non-alcoholic Fatty Liver Disease. Intern Med 2021;60(21):3391–9.

32. Idilman IS, Aniktar H, Idilman R, et al. Hepatic Steatosis: Quantification by Proton Density Fat Fraction with MR Imaging versus Liver Biopsy. Radiology 2013;267(3):767–75.

33. Colosimo S, Ravaioli F, Petroni ML, et al. Effects of antidiabetic agents on steatosis and fibrosis biomarkers in type 2 diabetes: A real-world data analysis. Liver Int 2021;41(4):731–42.

34. Gaborit B, Ancel P, Abdullah AE, et al. Effect of empagliflozin on ectopic fat stores and myocardial energetics in type 2 diabetes: the EMPACEF study. Cardiovasc Diabetol 2021;20(1):57.

35. Euh W, Lim S, Kim JW. Sodium-Glucose Cotransporter-2 Inhibitors Ameliorate Liver Enzyme Abnormalities in Korean Patients With Type 2 Diabetes Mellitus and Nonalcoholic Fatty Liver Disease. Front Endocrinol (Lausanne) 2021;12:613389.

36. Seko Y, Nishikawa T, Umemura A, et al. Efficacy and safety of canagliflozin in type 2 diabetes mellitus patients with biopsy-proven nonalcoholic steatohepatitis classified as stage 1-3 fibrosis. Diabetes Metab Syndr Obes 2018;11:835–43.

37. Marjot T, Green CJ, Charlton CA, et al. Sodium-glucose cotransporter 2 inhibition does not reduce hepatic steatosis in overweight, insulin-resistant patients without type 2 diabetes. JGH Open 2020;4(3):433–40.

38. Akuta N, Kawamura Y, Fujiyama S, et al. SGLT2 Inhibitor Treatment Outcome in Nonalcoholic Fatty Liver Disease Complicated with Diabetes Mellitus: The Long-term Effects on Clinical Features and Liver Histopathology. Intern Med 2020;59(16):1931–7.

39. Lai LL, Vethakkan SR, Nik Mustapha NR, et al. Empagliflozin for the Treatment of Nonalcoholic Steatohepatitis in Patients with Type 2 Diabetes Mellitus. Dig Dis Sci 2020;65(2):623–31.

40. Kern M, Klöting N, Mark M, et al. The SGLT2 inhibitor empagliflozin improves insulin sensitivity in db/db mice both as monotherapy and in combination with linagliptin. Metabolism 2016;65(2):114–23.

41. Xu L, Nagata N, Nagashimada M, et al. SGLT2 Inhibition by Empagliflozin Promotes Fat Utilization and Browning and Attenuates Inflammation and Insulin Resistance by Polarizing M2 Macrophages in Diet-induced Obese Mice. EBioMedicine 2017;20:137–49.

42. Kullmann S, Hummel J, Wagner R, et al. Empagliflozin Improves Insulin Sensitivity of the Hypothalamus in Humans With Prediabetes: A Randomized, Double-Blind, Placebo-Controlled, Phase 2 Trial. Diabetes Care 2022;45(2):398–406.

43. Latva-Rasku A, Honka MJ, Kullberg J, et al. The SGLT2 Inhibitor Dapagliflozin Reduces Liver Fat but Does Not Affect Tissue Insulin Sensitivity: A Randomized, Double-Blind, Placebo-Controlled Study With 8-Week Treatment in Type 2 Diabetes Patients. Diabetes Care 2019;42(5):931–7.

44. Yang Y, Zhao C, Ye Y, et al. Prospect of Sodium–Glucose Co-transporter 2 Inhibitors Combined With Insulin for the Treatment of Type 2 Diabetes. Front Endocrinol 2020;11.

45. Bonner C, Kerr-Conte J, Gmyr V, et al. Inhibition of the glucose transporter SGLT2 with dapagliflozin in pancreatic alpha cells triggers glucagon secretion. Nat Med 2015;21(5):512–7.

46. Salem V, Izzi-Engbeaya C, Coello C, et al. Glucagon increases energy expenditure independently of brown adipose tissue activation in humans. Diabetes Obes Metab 2016;18(1):72–81.

47. Makri ES, Goulas A, Polyzos SA. Sodium-glucose co-transporter 2 inhibitors in nonalcoholic fatty liver disease. Eur J Pharmacol 2021;907:174272.

48. Zhao P, Saltiel AR. From overnutrition to liver injury: AMP-activated protein kinase in nonalcoholic fatty liver diseases. J Biol Chem 2020;295(34):12279–89.

49. Porstmann T, Santos CR, Griffiths B, et al. SREBP activity is regulated by mTORC1 and contributes to Akt-dependent cell growth. Cell Metab 2008;8(3):224–36.

50. Laplante M, Sabatini DM. mTOR signaling in growth control and disease. Cell 2012;149(2):274–93.

51. Li Y, Chen Y. AMPK and Autophagy. Adv Exp Med Biol 2019;1206:85–108.

52. Kim J, Kundu M, Viollet B, et al. AMPK and mTOR regulate autophagy through direct phosphorylation of Ulk1. Nat Cell Biol 2011;13(2):132–41.

53. Ahmed BA, Ong FJ, Barra NG, et al. Lower brown adipose tissue activity is associated with non-alcoholic fatty liver disease but not changes in the gut microbiota. Cell Rep Med 2021;2(9):100397.

54. Han T, Fan Y, Gao J, et al. Sodium glucose cotransporter 2 inhibitor dapagliflozin depressed adiposity and ameliorated hepatic steatosis in high-fat diet induced obese mice. Adipocyte 2021;10(1):446–55.

55. Tilg H, Moschen AR. Evolution of inflammation in nonalcoholic fatty liver disease: The multiple parallel hits hypothesis. Hepatology 2010;52(5):1836–46.

56. Masarone M, Rosato V, Dallio M, et al. Role of Oxidative Stress in Pathophysiology of Nonalcoholic Fatty Liver Disease. Oxid Med Cell Longev 2018;2018:9547613.

57. Maejima Y. SGLT2 Inhibitors Play a Salutary Role in Heart Failure via Modulation of the Mitochondrial Function. Front Cardiovasc Med 2020;6.

58. Kanda T, Matsuoka S, Yamazaki M, et al. Apoptosis and non-alcoholic fatty liver diseases. World J Gastroenterol 2018;24(25):2661–72.

59. Raisova M, Hossini AM, Eberle J, et al. The Bax/Bcl-2 ratio determines the susceptibility of human melanoma cells to CD95/Fas-mediated apoptosis. J Invest Dermatol 2001;117(2):333–40.

60. Kruidering M, Evan GI. Caspase-8 in apoptosis: the beginning of "the end. IUBMB Life 2000;50(2):85–90.

61. Younossi ZM, Golabi P, de Avila L, et al. The global epidemiology of NAFLD and NASH in patients with type 2 diabetes: A systematic review and meta-analysis. J Hepatol 2019;71(4):793–801.

62. Lopaschuk GD, Verma S. Mechanisms of Cardiovascular Benefits of Sodium Glucose Co-Transporter 2 (SGLT2) Inhibitors: A State-of-the-Art Review. JACC Basic Transl Sci 2020;5(6):632–44.

SGLT2 Inhibitors and Safety in Older Patients

Rena Pollack, MD[a,b], Avivit Cahn, MD[a,c],*

KEYWORDS

- SGLT-2 inhibitors • Safety • Elderly • Volume depletion • Genital infections • Fractures
- Diabetic ketoacidosis • Hypoglycemia

KEY POINTS

- SGLT2 inhibitors (SGLT2i) are effective in the management of type 2 diabetes, with a reduction in heart failure hospitalizations and chronic kidney disease progression in older adults with and without diabetes.
- Treatment with SGLT2i in the elderly is generally safe.
- Risk of diabetic ketoacidosis is increased, although rare, and may be avoided by withholding medication during fasting or acute illness.
- Adverse events including volume depletion and hypoglycemia can potentially be avoided by proper patient selection, patient education and medication adjustment.
- Limited data exists regarding the risk of urinary tract infections, fractures, and amputations in the elderly treated with SGLT2i and routine monitoring is recommended.

INTRODUCTION

In recent years, the role of sodium glucose cotransporter 2 (SGLT-2) inhibitors (SGLT2i) has expanded beyond the treatment of diabetes alone to the prevention and treatment of heart failure and chronic kidney disease.[1–7] As the prevalence of these conditions increases exponentially with age, SGLT2i have important benefits in older patients.[8,9] Nonetheless, prescribing medications for the elderly (≥65 years) and particularly the very elderly (≥75 years) remains a challenge because they are at a greater risk for adverse drug events due to higher rates of polypharmacy, frailty, and cognitive impairment.[10] Although multiple programs have been proposed to reduce polypharmacy and adverse drug reactions in the elderly, underprescription of beneficial drugs remains an issue. Despite established benefits on mortality and quality of life, there is hesitation to prescribe such medications in the elderly due to multiple, although not always justified concerns.[11]

Because SGLT2i lower plasma glucose independent of insulin secretion, they are effective in any duration of disease.[12,13] Furthermore, they can be taken orally at any time of the day and have no known significant drug interactions.[14] The risk for hypoglycemia is minimal and the simplicity of administration has made this drug class an attractive option for the older adult population.[12] Still, there has been hesitancy in prescribing these agents for the elderly, mostly due to limited long-term data and concern regarding potential risks including volume depletion, acute kidney injury (AKI), diabetic ketoacidosis (DKA), amputations, and fractures.[15]

Accumulating evidence from randomized controlled trials (RCTs) and real-world studies (RWS) during the last decade have examined the safety of SGLT2i in older adults. Outcomes observed within age subgroups in the EMPA-REG OUTCOME, Dapagliflozin Effect on Cardiovascular Events–Thrombolysis in Myocardial

[a] The Faculty of Medicine, Hebrew University of Jerusalem, Jerusalem, Israel; [b] Department of Endocrinology and Metabolism, Hadassah-Hebrew University Medical Center, PO Box 12000, Jerusalem 91120, Israel; [c] Diabetes Unit, Department of Endocrinology and Metabolism, Hadassah-Hebrew University Medical Center, PO Box 12000, Jerusalem 91120, Israel
* Corresponding author.
E-mail address: avivit@hadassah.org.il

Heart Failure Clin 18 (2022) 635–643
https://doi.org/10.1016/j.hfc.2022.03.002

Infarction (DECLARE-TIMI 58), and Dapagliflozin and Prevention of Adverse Outcomes in Heart Failure (DAPA-HF) trials have demonstrated the efficacy and safety of empagliflozin and dapagliflozin in patients aged older than 65 years.[16-18] In this narrative review, we summarize the major safety issues raised regarding SGLT2i and review the available data on the safety of this novel therapeutic approach in the elderly and very elderly population.

SAFETY ISSUES ASSOCIATED WITH SGLT-2 INHIBITORS
Volume Depletion

SGLT2i lead to an increase in the urinary volume of up to 500 mL, potentially predisposing to volume depletion.[19] This concern has been mainly noted for the elderly or for those taking a concomitant diuretic, particularly loop diuretic therapy, although it has been proposed that SGLT2i might have a diuretic-sparing effect in patients with heart failure with reduced ejection fraction.[20] A meta-analysis of large RCTs noted an increased risk of volume depletion compared with standard of care (HR [95% CI] 1.14 [1.05, 1.24]).[21] This was mainly driven by an absolute increase in volume depletion events with canagliflozin in the Canagliflozin Cardiovascular Assessment Study (CANVAS) program and with dapagliflozin in the Dapagliflozin and Prevention of Adverse Outcomes in Chronic Kidney Disease (DAPA-CKD) trial, although a trend to an increased risk was observed in all trials.[21] In the DAPA-HF trial, volume depletion was slightly more common with dapagliflozin than with placebo in patients in the higher dose diuretic groups.[20] Therefore, adjusting the dose of loop diuretics in patients initiating SGLT2i may be appropriate for some patients.

In the large RCTs, elderly patients did not emerge as a particular risk group for volume depletion with SGLT2i, although some increase with empagliflozin in the very elderly was noted (Table 1).[16-18] Additionally, in a pooled safety analysis of RCTs of empagliflozin versus placebo, a slight increase of volume depletion-related adverse events was noted in patients aged 75 to 85 years treated with empagliflozin 10/25 mg versus placebo (5.9% vs 5.0%).[22] An increase in volume depletion events was also noted in a pooled safety analysis of phase 3 studies with canagliflozin in very elderly patients 75 years or older.[23] Adverse events related to volume depletion were noted in 2.6%, 4.9%, and 8.7% in the noncanagliflozin, 100 mg, and 300 mg canagliflozin groups, respectively.[23] Similarly, in a pooled analysis of phase 3 trials with ertugliflozin volume depletion was observed more frequently with ertugliflozin versus placebo in patients aged 65 years or older (1.3% in the nonertugliflozin group vs 2.2% and 3.3% in the ertugliflozin 5 and 15 mg groups, respectively).[24] The more frequent use of loop diuretics in the elderly, combined with a higher risk of frailty may predispose the elderly, and particularly the very elderly, to volume depletion events. Careful review of medication list, with consideration of dose reduction of other diuretics may be prudent when initiating SGLT2i in the frail elderly.

Acute Kidney Injury

The initial eGFR dip observed with SGLT2i, combined with concern regarding volume depletion events warranted further evaluation of whether these agents may predispose to AKI. However, both RCTs and observational data have consistently indicated lower rates of AKI with SGLT2i

Table 1
Volume depletion by age subgroups

Trial	Age	SGLT2i	Comparator
EMPA-REG OUTCOME[18]		Empagliflozin	Placebo
	<65	95/2596 (3.7%)	45/1297 (3.5%)
	65–<75	115/1667 (6.9%)	57/808 (7.1%)
	≥75	29/424 (6.8%)	13/228 (5.7%)
DECLARE-TIMI 58[17]		Dapagliflozin	Placebo
	<65	96/4626 (2.1%)	86/4619 (1.9%)
	65–<75	96/3411 (2.8%)	90/3395 (2.7%)
	≥75	21/537 (3.9%)	31/555 (5.6%)
DAPA-HF[16]		Dapagliflozin	Placebo
	<55	23/339 (6.8%)	14/295 (4.7%)
	55–64	36/610 (5.9%)	35/630 (5.6%)
	65–74	57/830 (6.9%)	57/886 (6.4%)
	≥75	62/589 (10.5%)	56/557 (10.1%)

versus comparators.[21,25,26] A reduction in AKI events with SGLT2i has been observed irrespective of age in the large RCTs as well as in observational studies (**Table 2**).[16–18,27] Importantly, multiple RCTs both in populations with and without diabetes demonstrated the important role of SGLT2i as renoprotective agents, across all age categories.[28]

Diabetic Ketoacidosis

DKA is a rare complication of type 2 diabetes, and its risk is doubled in patients treated with SGLT2i.[21,29,30] In the DAPA-HF and DAPA-CKD trials, DKA was not reported in patients without baseline diabetes.[5,31] In the DECLARE-TIMI 58 trial, the overall HR (95% CI) for DKA was 2.18 (1.10, 4.30) and no differential effect by age was noted in patients aged less than 65 years compared with patients aged 65 years or older (HR [95% CI] 2.05 [0.84, 5.03] vs 2.34 [0.82, 6.64]; interaction *P*-value 0.8538).[17] A meta-analysis of 39 RCTs, demonstrated an OR of 2.13 (1.38–3.27) for the development of DKA. The OR (95% CI) of DKA was 2.40 (1.46–3.95) in studies that included patients with a mean age of 60 years or older, and 0.64 (0.23–1.75) in studies that included patients with a mean age of less than 60 years (p-interaction 0.02). However, as this is not based on patient level data, it is difficult to interpret the clinical significance of these findings.[30] In a Scandinavian register-based cohort study, a doubling of the risk of ketoacidosis was noted in new users of SGLT2i compared with glucagon like peptide-1 (GLP-1) receptor agonists, and the risk seemed lower in patients aged 65 years or older compared with patients aged 35 to 65 years (HR [95% CI] 1.18 [0.38–3.69] vs

3.31 [1.17–9.34] respectively).[32] Overall, DKA is a rare event and reports to date have been restricted to patients with diabetes. In most cases, a predisposing factor may be identified including concomitant illness, fasting, dehydration, and reduced insulin dose.[29] Increasing awareness of DKA in these situations, withholding SGLT2i during acute illness, and careful reduction of insulin doses when initiating the treatment with SGLT2i may prevent many of these rare events.[33] The Professional Practice Committee of the American Diabetes Association recommends withholding SGLT2i 3 to 4 days before surgery to reduce the risk of perioperative complications.[34]

Hypoglycemia

SGLT2i reduce plasma glucose by promoting glucosuria in a noninsulin mediated mechanism, and the concomitant increase in endogenous glucose production prevents hypoglycemia.[35] In patients with diabetes, the propensity for causing hypoglycemia is largely dependent on background medications. Reduction of the daily dose of exogenous insulin or insulin secretagogue may prevent hypoglycemia, particularly in patients already close to their HbA1c target.[36] A meta-analysis of large RCTs with SGLT2i demonstrated a trend for reduction in the risk of severe hypoglycemia with SGLT2i (HR [95% CI] 0.86 [0.71, 1.03])—probably due to the higher use of insulin or sulfonylureas in the control arm required to control glycemia.[21] Notably, hypoglycemia did not occur in patients without diabetes in the DAPA-HF and DAPA-CKD trials.[5,31] In the EMPEROR-REDUCED (Empagliflozin Outcomes Trial in Heart Failure and a Reduced Ejection Fraction) trial, 7 versus 6 patients without baseline diabetes were

Table 2
Acute kidney injury by age subgroups

Trial	Age	SGLT2i	Comparator
EMPA-REG OUTCOME[18]		Empagliflozin	Placebo
	<65	16/2596 (0.6%)	16/1297 (1.2%)
	65–<75	19/1667 (1.1%)	14/808 (1.7%)
	≥75	10/424 (2.4%)	7/228 (3.1%)
DECLARE-TIMI 58[17]		Dapagliflozin	Placebo
	<65	58/4626 (1.3%)	80/4619 (1.7%)
	65–<75	56/3411 (1.6%)	73/3395 (2.2%)
	≥75	11/537 (2.0%)	22/555 (4.0%)
DAPA-HF[16]		Dapagliflozin	Placebo
	<55	3/339 (0.9%)	4/295 (1.4%)
	55–64	13/610 (2.1%)	9/630 (1.4%)
	65–74	19/830 (2.3%)	22/886 (2.5%)
	≥75	3/589 (0.5%)	30/557 (5.4%)

reported to have hypoglycemia with empagliflozin versus placebo, but a broader definition of hypoglycemia was used (plasma glucose value of ≤70 mg/dL or that required assistance).[6]

Elderly patients are at increased risk of hypoglycemia, in general, due to multiple factors including insulin deficiency, progressive renal insufficiency, and cognitive decline.[37] A pooled analysis of phase 3 studies with canagliflozin demonstrated overall low rates of severe hypoglycemia in patients aged 75 years or older treated with canagliflozin. In patients taking concomitant insulin, sulfonylureas, or meglitinides, rates were 5.5% in the noncanagliflozin arm versus 3.4% and 3.8% in the canagliflozin 100 mg and 300 mg arms, respectively.[23] In subgroup analyses of 3 large RCTs of SGLT2i by age, rates of major hypoglycemia increased with age, yet SGLT2i did not increase the risk of hypoglycemia at any age category (**Table 3**).[16–18] In the DECLARE-TIMI 58 study, major hypoglycemia was overall reduced (HR [95% CI] 0.68 [0.49–0.95]) with the reduction more prominent in the age group 65 years or older versus less than 65 years (HR 0.53 [95% CI 0.34, 0.83] vs 0.97 [0.58, 1.64], respectively; interaction P value 0.0896).[17]

Fractures

The risk of fractures increases markedly with age and diabetes itself is associated with an increased fracture risk.[38,39] Thus, bone health is extremely relevant when assessing new glucose lowering agent for elderly patients with diabetes. SGLT2i may indirectly disrupt calcium and phosphate homeostasis, contribute to weight loss and reduced blood pressure thus predisposing to falls and fractures.[38] Although an increased fracture risk was observed with canagliflozin in the CANVAS trial (HR [95% CI] 1.55 [1.21, 1.97]), this was not observed in the CANVAS-R (HR [95% CI] 0.86 [0.62, 1.19]), or Canagliflozin and Renal Endpoints in Diabetes with Established Nephropathy Clinical Evaluation (CREDENCE) trial (HR [95% CI] 0.98 [0.70, 1.37]) trials.[3,40] In a meta-analysis of large RCTs, the HR of fractures with SGLT2i versus standard of care was 1.07 (95% CI 0.99, 1.16).[21] No excess fracture risk was noted in the pooled analyses of trials from the development programs of ertugliflozin, empagliflozin, and dapagliflozin.[22,24,41] Additionally, a meta-analysis of 25 RCTs did not demonstrate an increased risk of fractures in those treated with metformin and an SGLT2i versus metformin monotherapy or other comparators.[42]

In subgroup analyses of 3 large RCT of SGLT2i by age, fracture rates increased with age, yet no interaction was noted between age group, drug, and fracture risk (interaction P-value 0.5245 for DECLARE TIMI 58, and not reported in other trials due to small numbers) (**Table 4**).[16–18] A comparable fracture risk was observed in a Korean retrospective cohort study of patients aged 65 years or older who initiated SGLT2i versus dipeptidyl peptidase-4 (DPP-4) inhibitors (HR [95% CI] 0.95 [0.88, 1.02]), with no increased risk observed in the subgroup of patients aged 75years or older.[43] Similarly, a Scandinavian register-based cohort study, which compared new users of SGLT2i versus GLP-1 receptor agonists did not indicate an increased fracture risk with SGLT2i in patients aged 65 years or older (HR [95% CI] 1.06 [0.82, 1.38]). Moreover, a population based new user cohort study, which included adults aged 65 years or older demonstrated no increased fracture risk with SGLT2i compared with GLP-1 RA or DPP-4

Table 3
Major hypoglycemia by age subgroups

Trial	Age	SGLT2i	Comparator
EMPA-REG OUTCOME[18]		Empagliflozin	Placebo
	<65	29/2596 (1.1%)	18/1297 (1.4%)
	65–<75	26/1667 (1.6%)	13/808 (1.6%)
	≥75	8/424 (1.9%)	5/228 (2.2%)
DECLARE-TIMI 58[17]		Dapagliflozin	Placebo
	<65	28/4626 (0.6%)	28/4619 (0.6%)
	65–<75	21/3411 (0.6%)	41/3395 (1.2%)
	≥75	9/537 (1.7%)	14/555 (2.5%)
DAPA-HF[16]		Dapagliflozin	Placebo
	<55	1/339 (0.3%)	0
	55–64	0	0
	65–74	2/830 (0.2%)	1/886 (0.1%)
	≥75	1/589 (0.2%)	3/557 (0.5%)

Table 4
Fractures by age subgroups

Trial	Age	SGLT2i	Comparator
EMPA-REG OUTCOME[18]		Empagliflozin	Placebo
	<65	45/2596 (3.5%)	81/1297 (3.1%)
	65–<75	76/1667 (4.6%)	35/808 (4.3%)
	≥75	22/424 (5.2%)	11/228 (4.8%)
DECLARE-TIMI 58[17]		Dapagliflozin	Placebo
	<65	205/4626 (4.4%)	200/4619 (4.3%)
	65–<75	212/3411 (6.2%)	208/3395 (6.1%)
	≥75	40/537 (7.4%)	33/555 (5.8%)
DAPA-HF[16]		Dapagliflozin	Placebo
	<55	1/339 (0.3%)	0
	55–64	11/610 (1.8%)	11/630 (1.7%)
	65–74	13/830 (1.6%)	24/886 (2.7%)
	≥75	24/589 (4.1%)	15/557 (2.7%)

inhibitors overall (HR [95% CI] 1.0 [0.8, 1,25] and 0.9 [0.73, 1.11], respectively), and in patients aged less than 75 or 75 years or older.[44] Overall, due to the low number of events reported, there is limited data in very elderly patients aged more than 75 years; however, the available data does seem reassuring.

Urinary Tract Infections

SGLT2i lead to increased glucosuria, thus altering the microbial flora of the genital region and potentially predisposing to urinary tract infections (UTI), although overall clinical data is inconclusive.[45] In a meta-analysis of large RCTs, the HR (95% CI) of UTI was 1.07 (0.99, 1.15).[21] A meta-analysis of 86 RCTs enrolling 50,880 patients noted no increase in UTIs compared with placebo (HR [95% CI] 1.03 [0.96, 1.11]) or active comparator (HR [95% CI] 1.08 [0.92, 1,25]).[46] A nationwide population based study in Korea demonstrated a marginal increase in UTIs in patients initiating SGLT2i versus DPP4 inhibitors (HR [95% CI] 1.05 [1.00, 1.11]).[43] Yet, no increased risk for outpatient UTIs was observed in a population based study in the United States in new users of SGLT2i versus DPP-4 inhibitors (HR [95% CI] 0.96 [0.89, 1.04]) or versus GLP-1 RA users (HR [95% CI] 0.91 [0.84, 0.99]), and severe UTI events were not increased as well.[47] There were no excess cases of Fournier gangrene, which was voiced as a concern with SGLT2i, with dapagliflozin in the DECLARE-TIMI 58 trial, and data was not reported in other large RCTs.[48] Nonetheless, it should be noted that many RCTs with SGLT2i excluded patients with recurrent UTI, and this may also be a potential confounder in observational studies.

Review of UTI risk by age did not demonstrate a predilection for UTIs with SGLT2i in the elderly or very elderly. In the DECLARE TIMI-58 trial, UTI (serious or leading to discontinuation of study drug) were not increased overall (HR [95% CI] 0.93 [0.73, 1.18]) and no age-based treatment interaction was demonstrated (interaction P-value 0.3066 for age categories <65 years, 65–<75 years, and ≥75 years).[4,17] Similarly, no increased risk of UTI was noted overall, in the elderly, or very elderly patients in the EMPA-REG study.[18] Pooled analysis of phase 3 trials with ertugliflozin did not show increased risk of UTI in patients aged less than 65 years or 65 years or older.[24] An observational study in Canada demonstrated no increased risk of UTI among new users of SGLT2i versus DPP-4 inhibitors in patients aged 66 years or older (HR [95% CI] 0.89 [0.78–1.0]). Thus, overall, although there may be a minimally increased risk of UTI with SGLT2i, the risk does not seem to increase with age.

Genital Tract Infections

The risk of genital infections is increased 3-fold to 5-fold in SGLT2i users due to increased concentrations of glucose in the genitourinary tract.[49] In a meta-analysis of large RCTs, SGLT2i increased the risk of genital infections (HR [95% CI] 3.75 [3.0, 4.67]).[21] Similarly, a meta-analysis of 86 RCTs enrolling 50,880 patients, also noted a similar increase in genital infections with the use of SGLT2i versus placebo (HR [95% CI] 3.37 [2.89, 3.93]) or active comparator (HR [95% CI] 3.89 [3.14, 4.82]).[46] Female sex and history of prior genital infection seem to be the strongest predictors for genital tract infections among users of SGLT2i.[50]

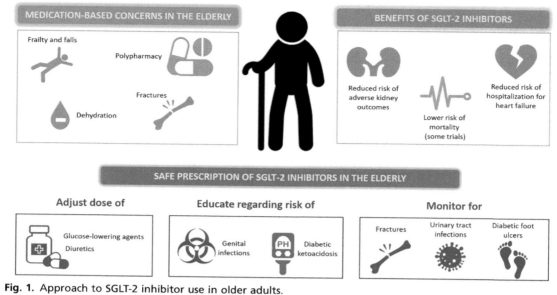

Fig. 1. Approach to SGLT-2 inhibitor use in older adults.

Elderly patients are not at excess risk of developing genital infections with SGLT2i. There was no age-based treatment interaction of serious genital infections or genital infections leading to drug discontinuation with dapagliflozin versus placebo in the DECLARE-TIMI 58 trial (HR [95% CI] 6.07 [2.56, 14.38] in patients aged younger than 65 years and HR [95% CI] 12.86 [3.98, 41.62] in patients aged ≥65 years; interaction P-value 0.3116).[17] Similarly, in the EMPA-REG OUTCOME trial, an excess risk of genital infections was reported across all age groups.[18]

Amputations

A nearly 2-fold increase in rate of amputations with canagliflozin versus placebo was observed in the CANVAS program leading to increased vigilance for this potential complication with SGLT2i.[3] Nonetheless, an excess risk of amputation was not observed in any of the other large RCTs with SGLT2i, or in the CREDENCE trial of renal outcomes with canagliflozin versus placebo.[21] A United States cohort study indicated a small increase in the rate of amputation in new users of canagliflozin versus GLP1-RA in patients aged 65 years or older with baseline cardiovascular disease (HR [95% CI] 1.73 [1.30, 2.29]).[51] Additional observation studies have shown mixed results.[32,52,53]

The increased risk of amputations is more relevant to the elderly, who are more likely to suffer from peripheral arterial disease (PAD) and use diuretics, because it has been proposed that volume depletion may predispose to reduced perfusion in the distal lower extremities.[54] However, no increased risk of amputation was observed in the DECLARE-TIMI 58 trial, or in the DAPA-HF trial, overall, and by age subgroups.[16,17] Additionally, a meta-analysis of large RCTs did not demonstrate an increased risk of amputation in elderly patients aged 65 years or older (HR [95% CI] 1.23 [0.59, 2.56]).[55] Although overall data is encouraging, careful observation of elderly patients with PAD receiving SGLT2i is recommended.

SUMMARY

SGLT2i are a valuable treatment option in older adults given their efficacy in the management of type 2 diabetes as well as their reduction in adverse cardiovascular and renal outcomes. Evidence from large RCTs and RWS have demonstrated long-term safety and tolerability overall, and in the elderly and very elderly population. Adverse events associated with SGLT2i are impacted by patient frailty, comorbidities, and concomitant medication use and therefore, must be thoroughly evaluated before initiating SGLT2i treatment. Common adverse events can be minimized by appropriate patient selection, patient education, and early recognition of symptoms (**Fig. 1**). When initiating therapy in the frail elderly population, the established benefits of these agents on diabetes, cardiovascular and renal diseases should be weighed against the potential risks.

CLINICS CARE POINTS

- SGLT2i have demonstrated efficacy in the management of type 2 diabetes as well as heart failure and chronic kidney disease in older adults with and without diabetes.

- The risk of hypoglycemia in the elderly is low unless there is concomitant administration with insulin or an insulin secretagogue.

- Volume depletion and hypotension may occur in susceptible individuals. Adjustment of concomitant therapies, particularly loop diuretics, should be performed to reduce risk.

- The risk of DKA is rare, and not particularly increased in the elderly compared with younger adults. Proper patient selection and patient education can minimize risk.

- Genital tract infections are common irrespective of age, however, are generally mild.

- The increased risk of UTI with SGLT2i use is inconclusive and caution should be exercised in initiating treatment in the elderly with recurrent UTI given limited data.

- Although initial studies suggested increased fracture risk and rate of amputations in patients receiving canagliflozin, these risks have not been reproduced in additional RCTs including older adults treated with SGLT2i. Nonetheless, routine bone mineral density monitoring and careful observation of elderly patients with PAD is recommended.

DISCLOSURE

R. Pollack has no conflicts of interest to disclose. A. Cahn reports grants and personal fees from AstraZeneca and Novo Nordisk and personal fees from Boehringer Ingelheim, Eli Lilly, Pfizer, and Medial Early-Sign.

REFERENCES

1. Zinman B, Wanner C, et al. Empagliflozin, cardiovascular outcomes, and mortality in type 2 diabetes. N Engl J Med 2015;373(22):2117–28.

2. Wanner C, Inzucchi SE, Lachin JM, et al. Empagliflozin and Progression of Kidney Disease in Type 2 Diabetes. N Engl J Med 2016;375(4):323–34.

3. Neal B, Perkovic V, Mahaffey KW, et al. Canagliflozin and cardiovascular and renal events in type 2 diabetes. N Engl J Med 2017;377(7):644–57.

4. Wiviott SD, Raz I, Bonaca MP, et al. Dapagliflozin and cardiovascular outcomes in type 2 diabetes. N Engl J Med 2019;380(4):347–57.

5. McMurray J, Solomon S, Inzucchi S, et al. Dapagliflozin in patients with heart failure and reduced ejection fraction. N Engl J Med 2019;381(21): 1995–2008.

6. Packer M, Anker SD, Butler J, et al. Cardiovascular and renal outcomes with empagliflozin in heart failure. N Engl J Med 2020;383(15):1413–24.

7. Anker SD, Butler J, Filippatos G, et al. Effect of empagliflozin on cardiovascular and renal outcomes in patients with heart failure by baseline diabetes status: results from the EMPEROR-REDUCED trial. Circulation 2021;143(4):337–49.

8. Groenewegen A, Rutten FH, Mosterd A, et al. Epidemiology of heart failure. Eur J Heart Fail 2020;22(8): 1342–56.

9. International Diabetes Federation. IDF Diabetes Atlas, 10th edn Brussels, Belgium. 2021. Available at: https://diabetesatlas.org/idfawp/resource-files/2021/07/IDF_Atlas_10th_Edition_2021.pdf. Accessed April 1, 2022.

10. Zazzara MB, Palmer K, Liborio Vetrano D, et al. Adverse drug reactions in older adults: a narrative review of the literature. Eur Geriatr Med 1999;12: 463–73.

11. Lombardi F, Paoletti L, Carrieri B, et al. Underprescription of medications in older adults: causes, consequences and solutions-a narrative review. Eur Geriatr Med 2021;12(3):453–62.

12. Abdul-Ghani MA, DeFronzo RA, Norton L. Novel hypothesis to explain why SGLT2 inhibitors inhibit only 30-50% of filtered glucose load in humans. Diabetes 2013;62(10):3324–8.

13. Zhang L, Feng Y, List J, et al. Dapagliflozin treatment in patients with different stages of type 2 diabetes mellitus: effects on glycaemic control and body weight. Diabetes Obes Metab 2010;12(6): 510–6.

14. Scheen AJ. Pharmacokinetics, pharmacodynamics and clinical use of SGLT2 inhibitors in patients with type 2 diabetes mellitus and chronic kidney disease. Clin Pharmacokinet 2015;54(7):691–708.

15. FDA. U.S. Food and Drug Administration; Drug Safety Communications. 2018. Available at: https://www.fda.gov/drugs/postmarket-drug-safety-information-patients-and-providers/sodium-glucose-cotransporter-2-sglt2-inhibitors. Accessed April 1, 2022.

16. Martinez FA, Serenelli M, Nicolau JC, et al. Efficacy and safety of dapagliflozin in heart failure with reduced ejection fraction according to age: insights from DAPA-HF. Circulation 2020;141(1):100–11.

17. Cahn A, Mosenzon O, Wiviott SD, et al. Efficacy and safety of dapagliflozin in the elderly: analysis from the DECLARE-TIMI 58 study. Diabetes Care 2020; 43(2):468–75.

18. Monteiro P, Bergenstal RM, Toural E, et al. Efficacy and safety of empagliflozin in older patients in the

EMPA-REG OUTCOME® trial. Age Ageing 2019; 48(6):859–66.

19. Mordi NA, Mordi IR, Singh JS, et al. Renal and cardiovascular effects of SGLT2 inhibition in combination with loop diuretics in patients with type 2 diabetes and chronic heart failure: the RECEDE-CHF trial. Circulation 2020;142:1713–24.

20. Jackson AM, Dewan P, Anand IS, et al. Dapagliflozin and diuretic use in patients with heart failure and reduced ejection fraction in DAPA-HF. Circulation 2020;1040–54.

21. Qiu M, Ding LL, Zhang M, et al. Safety of four SGLT2 inhibitors in three chronic diseases: a meta-analysis of large randomized trials of SGLT2 inhibitors. Diabetes Vasc Dis Res 2021;18(2):1–3.

22. Kinduryte Schorling O, Clark D, Zwiener I, et al. Pooled safety and tolerability analysis of empagliflozin in patients with type 2 diabetes mellitus. Adv Ther 2020;37(8):3463–84.

23. Sinclair AJ, Bode B, Harris S, et al. Efficacy and safety of canagliflozin in individuals aged 75 and older with type 2 diabetes mellitus: a pooled analysis. Wiley Online Libr 2016;64(3):543–52.

24. Pratley R, Dagogo-Jack S, Charbonnel B, et al. Efficacy and safety of ertugliflozin in older patients with type 2 diabetes: a pooled analysis of phase III studies. Wiley Online Libr 2020;22(12):2276–86.

25. Cahn A, Melzer-Cohen C, Diabetes RP. Obesity undefined, 2019 undefined. Acute renal outcomes with sodium-glucose co-transporter-2 inhibitors: real-world data analysis. Wiley Online Libr 2018;21(2):340–8.

26. Menne J, Dumann E, Haller H, et al. Acute kidney injury and adverse renal events in patients receiving SGLT2-inhibitors: a systematic review and meta-analysis. PLOS Med 2019;16(12):e1002983.

27. Iskander C, Cherney DZ, Clemens KK, et al. Use of sodium-glucose cotransporter-2 inhibitors and risk of acute kidney injury in older adults with diabetes: a population-based cohort study. CMAJ 2020; 192(14):E351–60.

28. Scheen AJ. Sodium–glucose cotransporter type 2 inhibitors for the treatment of type 2 diabetes mellitus. Nat Rev Endocrinol 2020;16(10):556–77.

29. Cahn A, Raz I, Bonaca M, et al. Safety of dapagliflozin in a broad population of patients with type 2 diabetes: analyses from the DECLARE-TIMI 58 study. Diabetes Obes Metab 2020;22(8):1357–68.

30. Liu J, Li L, Li S, et al. Sodium-glucose co-transporter-2 inhibitors and the risk of diabetic ketoacidosis in patients with type 2 diabetes: a systematic review and meta-analysis of randomized controlled trials. Diabetes Obes Metab 2020;22(9):1619–27.

31. Heerspink HJL, Stefánsson BV, Correa-Rotter R, et al. Dapagliflozin in patients with chronic kidney disease. N Engl J Med 2020;383(15):1436–46.

32. Ueda P, Svanström H, Melbye M, et al. Sodium glucose cotransporter 2 inhibitors and risk of serious adverse events: Nationwide register based cohort study. BMJ 2018;363:4365.

33. Rosenstock J, Ferrannini E. Euglycemic diabetic ketoacidosis: A predictable, detectable, and preventable safety concern with sglt2 inhibitors. Diabetes Care 2015;38(9):1638–42.

34. 16. Diabetes care in the hospital: standards of medical care in diabetes—2022. Diabetes Care 2022; 45(Supplement_1):S244–53.

35. Kuhre RE, Deacon CF, Wewer Albrechtsen NJ, et al. Do sodium-glucose co-transporter-2 inhibitors increase plasma glucagon by direct actions on the alpha cell? And does the increase matter for the associated increase in endogenous glucose production? Diabetes Obes Metab 2021;23(9):2009–19.

36. Scheen AJ. Careful use to minimize adverse events of oral antidiabetic medications in the elderly. Expert Opin Pharmacother 2021;22(16):2149–65.

37. Committee ADAPP. 13. older adults: standards of medical care in diabetes—2022. Diabetes Care 2022;45(Supplement_1):S195–207.

38. Farooqui KJ, Mithal A, Kerwen AK, et al. Type 2 diabetes and bone fragility- An under-recognized association. Diabetes Metab Syndr Clin Res Rev 2021; 15(3):927–35.

39. Schwartz AV, Vittinghoff E, Bauer DC, et al. Association of BMD and FRAX score with risk of fracture in older adults with type 2 diabetes. JAMA 2011; 305(21):2184–92.

40. Perkovic V, Jardine MJ, Neal B, et al. Canagliflozin and renal outcomes in type 2 diabetes and nephropathy. N Engl J Med 2019;380(24):2295–306.

41. Jabbour S, Seufert J, Scheen A, et al. Dapagliflozin in patients with type 2 diabetes mellitus: a pooled analysis of safety data from phase IIb/III clinical trials. Diabetes Obes Metab 2018;20(3):620–8.

42. Qian BB, Chen Q, Li L, et al. Association between combined treatment with SGLT2 inhibitors and metformin for type 2 diabetes mellitus on fracture risk: a meta-analysis of randomized controlled trials. Osteoporos Int 2020;31(12):2313–20.

43. Han SJ, Ha KH, Lee N, et al. Effectiveness and safety of sodium-glucose co-transporter-2 inhibitors compared with dipeptidyl peptidase-4 inhibitors in older adults with type 2 diabetes: a nationwide population-based study. Diabetes Obes Metab 2021;23(3):682–91.

44. Zhuo M, Hawley CE, Paik JM, et al. Association of sodium-glucose cotransporter–2 inhibitors with fracture risk in older adults with type 2 diabetes. JAMA Netw Open 2021;4(10):e2130762.

45. Geerlings S, Fonseca V, Castro-Diaz D, et al. Genital and urinary tract infections in diabetes: impact of pharmacologically-induced glucosuria. Diabetes Res Clin Pract 2014;103(3):373–81.

46. Puckrin R, Saltiel MP, Reynier P, et al. SGLT-2 inhibitors and the risk of infections: a systematic review

and meta-analysis of randomized controlled trials. Acta Diabetol 2018;55(5):503–14.

47. Dave CV, Schneeweiss S, Kim D, et al. Sodium-glucose cotransporter-2 inhibitors and the risk for severe urinary tract infections. Ann Intern Med 2019;171(4):248–56.

48. Scheen AJ. An update on the safety of SGLT2 inhibitors. Expert Opin Drug Saf 2019;18(4):295–311.

49. Lega IC, Bronskill SE, Campitelli Msc MA, et al. Sodium glucose cotransporter 2 inhibitors and risk of genital mycotic and urinary tract infection: a population-based study of older women and men with diabetes. Wiley Online Libr 2019;21(11):2394–404.

50. McGovern AP, Hogg M, Shields BM, et al. Risk factors for genital infections in people initiating SGLT2 inhibitors and their impact on discontinuation. BMJ Open Diabetes Res Care 2020;8(1):e001238.

51. Fralick M, Kim SC, Schneeweiss S, et al. Risk of amputation with canagliflozin across categories of age and cardiovascular risk in three US nationwide databases: cohort study. BMJ 2020;370:2812.

52. Chang HY, Singh S, Mansour O, et al. Association between sodium-glucose cotransporter 2 inhibitors and lower extremity amputation among patients with type 2 diabetes. JAMA Intern Med 2018;178(9):1242–8.

53. Yu OHY, Dell'Aniello S, Shah BR, et al. Sodium–glucose cotransporter 2 inhibitors and the risk of below-knee amputation: a multicenter observational study. Diabetes Care 2020;43(10):2444–52.

54. Alshnbari A, Alkharaiji M, Anyanwagu U, et al. Diuretics and risk of lower extremity amputation amongst patients with insulin-treated type 2 diabetes–exploring the mechanism of possible sodium glucose co-transporter 2 inhibitor induced risk of lower extremity amputations. Curr Med Res Opin 2020;36(12):1985–9.

55. Huang CY, Lee JK. Sodium-glucose co-transporter-2 inhibitors and major adverse limb events: a trial-level meta-analysis including 51 713 individuals. Diabetes Obes Metab 2020;22(12):2348–55.

Sodium Glucose Cotransporter 2 Inhibitors, Amputation Risk, and Fracture Risk

Clare Arnott, MBBS(Hons), PhD[a,b,c,]*, Robert A. Fletcher, MSc[a], Bruce Neal, MB ChB, PhD[a,d]

KEYWORDS

- SGLT2 inhibitors • Meta-analysis • Amputation • Fracture

KEY POINTS

- In the 11 cardiovascular and renal outcome trials of sodium glucose cotransporter 2 (SGLT2) inhibition done in a broad range of patients, active treatment does not increase the risk of amputation or fracture.
- No patient subgroup, defined by age, sex, disease history, or other patient characteristic, has been identified as at higher risk of amputation or fracture caused by SGLT2 inhibitor treatment.
- Isolated elevations in amputation and fracture risks associated with canagliflozin treatment in the CANagliflozin cardioVascular Assessment Study program cannot be explained by participant, trial, or drug factors and are likely chance findings.

INTRODUCTION

The first sodium glucose cotransporter 2 (SGLT2) inhibitor, canagliflozin, was approved by the Food and Drug Administration (FDA) in the United States in 2013 as an oral hypoglycemic agent for the treatment of type 2 diabetes (T2D). Initial indications were for those with high-risk disease as second or third line "add-on" therapy.[1–3] Since then the broad cardiovascular (CV), kidney, and mortality benefits of this drug class across multiple target populations have become apparent based on the findings of several landmark cardiovascular outcome trials and renal outcome trials.[4–7]

In those with T2D and high CV risk or established CV disease, SGLT2 inhibitors reduce hospitalization for heart failure by more than 30%, as well as providing significant reductions in CV death, major adverse cardiac events (MACE:

nonfatal myocardial infarction (MI), nonfatal stoke, and CV death), all-cause mortality and adverse renal events.[8,9] These benefits have now been shown to extend to those with chronic kidney disease (CKD),[10] those with heart failure with reduced ejection fraction (HFrEF)[11,12] and those with heart failure with preserved ejection fraction, irrespective of the presence of T2D.[13] Importantly, these benefits seem to be a class effect, with no clear evidence to support heterogeneity in the effects of the different compounds.[14,15]

These data have led to updates of T2D and heart failure guidelines worldwide to incorporate SGLT2 inhibitors into treatment algorithms. For example, the American Diabetes Association revised their T2D guidelines in 2021 to recommend SGLT2 inhibitors in those with established atherosclerotic CV disease or CKD "irrespective of A1C levels" to "reduce the risk of major adverse CV events

[a] The George Institute for Global Health, University of New South Wales, Level 5, 1 King Street, Newtown, Sydney 2042, Australia; [b] Department of Cardiology, Royal Prince Alfred Hospital, Sydney, Australia; [c] Sydney Medical School, University of Sydney, New South Wales, Australia; [d] Department of Epidemiology and Biostatistics, Imperial College London, London, United Kingdom
* Corresponding author. The George Institute for Global Health, University of New South Wales, Level 5, 1 King Street, Newtown, Sydney 2042, Australia.
E-mail address: carnott@georgeinstitute.org.au

Heart Failure Clin 18 (2022) 645–654
https://doi.org/10.1016/j.hfc.2022.03.008
1551-7136/22/© 2022 Elsevier Inc. All rights reserved.

and heart failure hospitalization."[16] Similarly, in 2021, the European Society of Cardiology added SGLT2 inhibitors to their guideline recommendations for the treatment of chronic HFrEF.[17] As for every new therapy, the clinical benefits need to be weighed against potential risks. Indeed, there has been some clinical inertia in the prescription of SGLT2 inhibitors with one US study suggesting only 33% of eligible T2D patients are currently receiving them.[18] This is thought to be at least partially due to concerns about serious side effects.

Although SGLT2 inhibitors reduce total serious adverse events, they are known to increase the risk of genital mycotic infections and hypotension.[8] Whether they increase the risk of amputation and fracture, however, has been in contention since early signals of concern from the CANVAS (CANagliflozin cardioVascular Assessment Study) Program investigating the effects of canagliflozin.[4]

In this review, we evaluate the available data on amputation and fracture risk for the different SGLT2 inhibitors within the drug class and for a range of different patient populations. We review postulated physiologic mechanisms linking the drug class to amputation and fracture and draw conclusions about the likelihood that these are real side effects of SGLT2 inhibitors.

AMPUTATION
Canagliflozin and Amputation Risk

Initial concerns regarding a possible effect of SGLT2 inhibitors on amputation were first identified following publication of the CANVAS program.[4] This consisted of 2 trials (CANVAS and CANVAS- Renal [CANVAS-R]) that reported on the CV benefits of the SGLT2 inhibitor canagliflozin in 10,142 participants with T2D and high CV risk. Although those assigned to active therapy achieved important cardiorenal protection, those treated with canagliflozin had a 97% relative increase in amputation risk (Hazard Ratio (HR) 1.97; 95% CI 1.41, 2.75) as compared with the placebo arm. A signal that seemed consistent across sex, age, and other key participant subgroups (**Fig. 1**). When assessing the breakdown of amputation types, both minor amputation (HR 1.94, 95% CI 1.31, 2.88) and major amputation (HR 2.03, 95% CI 1.08, 3.82) were significantly elevated with canagliflozin treatment,[19] and this finding resulted in canagliflozin receiving a "boxed warning" from the FDA in the United States in 2017.[1]

Concurrently, the CREDENCE (Canagliflozin and Renal Events in Diabetes with Established Nephropathy Clinical Evaluation) trial[7] was recruiting participants with T2D and albuminuric CKD to a renal outcomes trial of canagliflozin versus placebo. Following publication of the CANVAS program amputation findings a protocol amendment was made, three-quarters of the way through recruitment, to exclude enrollment of participants with a history of atraumatic amputation. Despite this protocol update, the final CREDENCE trial population (4401 participants) had a greater proportion of patients with a baseline history of amputation than the CANVAS program (5.3% vs 2.3%) and a higher amputation event rate (CREDENCE 3.0% annual event rate vs CANVAS 1.8%).[19] Overall amputation risk, however, was not increased by canagliflozin treatment in the CREDENCE trial (HR 1.11, 95% CI 0.79, 1.55) and neither was the risk of minor (HR 1.15, 95% CI 0.77, 1.69) nor major amputation (HR 0.78%, 95% 0.45, 1.36). The absence of harm in CREDENCE was observed across all participant subgroups defined by baseline characteristics, as well as before and after the protocol amendment. Meta-analysis of the 2 trials showed no overall amputation risk with canagliflozin, but there was significant heterogeneity (I2 = 82%, p heterogeneity = 0.018) between the findings for the CANVAS program and the CREDENCE trial (**Fig. 2**). A thorough analysis of both trials failed to identify a participant or trial factor to explain this between trial heterogeneity, and suggested chance as the most plausible explanation for the amputation signal identified in the CANVAS program.[19]

The CANVAS program and the CREDENCE trial are the only large-scale randomized clinical outcome trials done using canagliflozin, and although substantive in size and well powered to address their primary outcomes, the capacity to fully explore the associations with infrequent serious adverse events is limited. So called "real world" nonrandomized data have been used in an effort to better understand the most likely effects of canagliflozin on amputation risk. Analyses of these datasets report varied signals-from increased amputation risk with canagliflozin in the EASEL study,[20] modestly increased risk in those older than 65 years or those with CV disease in a US nationwide dataset,[21] to no increase in risk in either the OBSERVE-4D meta-analysis,[22] or another large US cohort of greater than 3 million adults with T2D.[23] The key challenge with these datasets is that although they are often substantial in size, they are observational in nature and regardless of the degree of sophistication of the analytical approaches used, residual confounding cannot be excluded. The diversity of the "real world" findings for amputation risk with

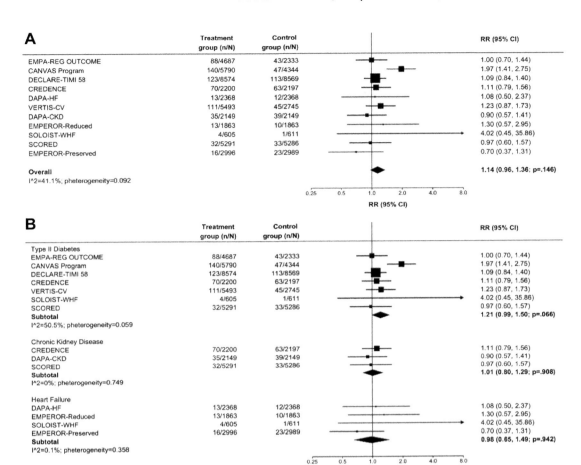

Fig. 1. Amputation risk overall (*A*) and by trial population (*B*). Meta-analysis using HR and RR when HR unavailable. Performed using random-effects meta-analysis using R. HR used: EMPA-REG Outcome, CANVAS, DECLARE-TIMI 58, CREDENCE. RR used: DAPA-HF, VERTIS-CV, DAPA-CKD, EMPEROR-Reduced, SOLOIST-WHF, SCORED, EMPEROR-Preserved.

canagliflozin highlight this problem, and the "real world" data analyses do little to inform our interpretation of the randomized data. More helpful in understanding the likely risk of amputation with SGLT2 inhibition are analyses of the many other large-scale randomized trials of SGLT2 inhibitors, with comparison of the effects on amputation, and other outcomes, across the totality of the evidence base.

All sodium glucose cotransporter 2 inhibitors and amputation risk

Including the 2 canagliflozin studies, there are 11 large-scale randomized trials (sample sizes: 1222–17,160; **Table 1**) that have been conducted using SGLT2 inhibitors in a range of patients with T2D, CKD, and heart failure (including both those with reduced and preserved ejection fraction).

These trials have tested the compounds empagliflozin (3 trials), dapagliflozin (3 trials), canagliflozin (2 trials), ertugliflozin (1 trial), and sotagliflozin (2 trials) (see **Table 1**). A total of 1074 amputation events have been recorded across these studies.

An updated meta-analysis of the risks of amputation in these 11 studies (using HRs or risk ratios [RR] dependent on available data) done for this report using a random effects model identified no increase in overall amputation risk across all studies (RR 1.14; 95% CI 0.96, 1.36). There was moderate evidence of heterogeneity in the individual study results (I2 = 41%, p heterogeneity = 0.092) that seemed to be driven by the CANVAS program result (see **Fig. 1**, Panel A). When the analysis was replicated following exclusion of the CANVAS program, the RR was 1.06 (95% CI 0.93, 1.21) with no evidence of heterogeneity (I2 = 0%, p heterogeneity = 0.84).

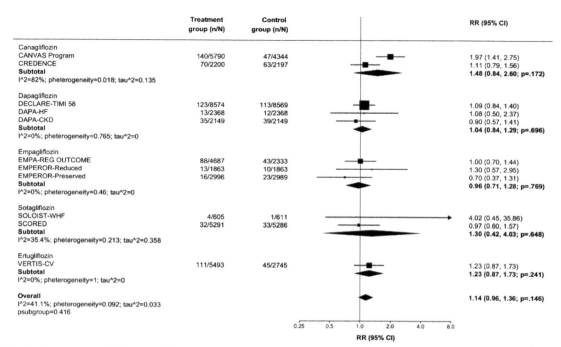

Fig. 2. Amputation risk by specific SGLT2 inhibitor compound. Meta-analysis using HR and RR when HR unavailable performed using random-effects meta-analysis using R. Test for moderators in the subgroup analysis was computed by mixed-effects meta-regression with Knapp-Hartung adjustment. HR used: EMPA-REG Outcome, CANVAS, DECLARE-TIMI 58, CREDENCE. RR used: DAPA-HF, VERTIS-CV, DAPA-CKD, EMPEROR-Reduced, SOLOIST-WHF, SCORED, EMPEROR-Preserved.

In terms of the other compounds, dapagliflozin has not been associated with an increased amputation risk as compared with placebo overall (335 events, RR 1.04; 95% CI 0.84, 1.29) or separately in those with T2D (RR 1.09; 95% CI 0.84, 1.40),[5] those with HFrEF (RR 1.08; 95% CI 0.50, 2.37),[11] or those with CKD (RR 0.90, 95% CI 0.57, 1.41).[10] Similarly, no association between empagliflozin and amputation has been identified overall (193 events, RR 0.96; 95% CI 0.71, 1.28) or in those with T2D (RR 1.00; 95% CI 0.70, 1.44),[6] HFrEF (RR 1.30; 95% CI 0.57, 2.95),[12] or heart failure with preserved ejection fraction (RR 0.70; 95% CI 0.37, 1.31).[13] Null effects were also observed for sotagliflozin in a mixed T2D and CKD population (RR 0.97; 95% CI 0.60, 1.57),[24] but the SOLOIST-worsening heart failure (SOLOIST-WHF) study[25] of sotaglflozin in T2D and heart failure reported too few amputation events to draw meaningful conclusions (4 events in the active arm, 1 event in the placebo arm). The single study of ertugliflozin done in a T2D population reported no increase in amputation with active treatment (156 events, RR 1.23; 95% CI 0.87, 1.73)[26] (see **Fig. 2**).

In meta-analyses assessing amputation risk in subgroups defined by the type of population included in the trial, there was no evidence that the risk of amputation with SGLT2 inhibition was increased in populations defined by T2D (RR 1.21; 95% CI 0.99, 1.57), CKD (RR 1.01; 95% CI 0.80, 1.29) or heart failure (RR 0.98; 95% CI 0.65, 1.49) (see **Fig. 1**B). There was moderate heterogeneity of the individual trial results for the T2D subset, which included the CANVAS program but not for those with CKD or heart failure.

Potential mechanisms for causation of amputation with sodium glucose cotransporter 2 inhibition

Those with T2D are at a heightened risk of peripheral arterial disease and amputation, as are those with CKD and heart failure.[27] The CANVAS program, the CREDENCE trial, and most of other large-scale studies of SGLT2 inhibitors would have all been expected a priori to accrue a relatively large number of amputation events during trial follow-up as a consequence of the baseline participant risks. However, the increased treatment-related amputation risk with canagliflozin identified in the CANVAS program was entirely unexpected. In general, the effects of SGLT2 inhibitors on intermediate risks such as glycemia

Table 1
Cardiovascular and renal outcome studies for SGLT2 inhibitor drug class

Completed Trial	Intervention	Study Size (n)	Population	Primary Outcome
EMPA-REG OUTCOME[6]	Empagliflozin	7020	T2D	MACE
CANVAS program[4]	Canagliflozin	10,142	T2D	MACE
DECLARE-TIMI 58[5]	Dapagliflozin	17,160	T2D	MACE
CREDENCE[7]	Canagliflozin	4401	T2D and CKD	Composite of ESKD, doubling of serum creatinine, renal, or CV death
DAPA-HF[11]	Dapagliflozin	4744	HF	Worsening HF (hospitalization or an urgent visit resulting in intravenous therapy for HF) or CV death
VERTIS-CV[26]	Ertugliflozin	8246	T2D	MACE
DAPA-CKD[10]	Dapagliflozin	4304	CKD	Composite of $\geq$50% sustained decline in eGFR, ESKD, renal, or CV death
EMPEROR-Reduced[12]	Empagliflozin	3730	HF	CV death or hospitalization for worsening HF
SOLOIST-WHF[25]	Sotagliflozin	1222	T2D and HF	CV death and hospitalizations and urgent visits for HF
SCORED[24]	Sotagliflozin	10,584	T2D and CKD	CV death, hospitalizations for HF, and urgent visits for HF
EMPEROR-Preserved[13]	Empagliflozin	2997	HF	CV death or hospitalization for worsening HF

Abbreviations: CANVAS program, Canagliflozin Cardiovascular Assessment Study Program; CREDENCE, Canagliflozin and renal events in diabetes with established nephropathy clinical evaluation; DAPA-CKD, Dapagliflozin and prevention of adverse outcomes in chronic kidney disease; DAPA-HF, Dapagliflozin and prevention of adverse outcomes in heart failure; DECLARE-TIMI 58, Dapagliflozin Effect on Cardiovascular Events–Thrombolysis in Myocardial Infarction 58; EMPA-REG OUTCOME, Empagliflozin Cardiovascular Outcome Event Trial in Type 2 Diabetes Mellitus Patients; EMPEROR-Preserved, empagliflozin Outcome Trial in Patients with Chronic Heart Failure with Preserved Ejection Fraction; EMPEROR-Reduced, Empagliflozin Outcome Trial in Patients with Chronic Heart Failure and a Reduced Ejection Fraction; SCORED, Effect of Sotagliflozin on Cardiovascular and Renal Events in Patients with Type 2 Diabetes and Moderate Renal Impairment Who Are at Cardiovascular Risk; SOLOIST-WHF, Effect of Sotagliflozin on Cardiovascular Events in Patients with Type 2 Diabetes Post Worsening Heart Failure; VERTIS-CV, Evaluation of ertugliflozin efficacy and safety cardiovascular outcomes trial.

would have been anticipated to reduce, not increase, the risk of amputation, and the signal for amputation risk was entirely unforeseen.

Subsequent to reporting of the CANVAS program findings, there has been a great deal of speculation regarding potential mechanisms. A "hemodynamic hypothesis" whereby hypotension caused by diuresis-driven volume depletion and body weight reduction may precipitate an increase in amputation events due to hypoperfusion was a primary mechanism investigated. A recent systematic review included a meta-regression of participant factors associated with amputation risk and identified an association of reductions in body weight and systolic blood pressure with amputation, lending some support to this possibility.[28] However, other agents that precipitate much larger reductions in body weight (eg, glucagon-like peptide 1 receptor agonists) and blood pressure

(antihypertensives) are not associated with an increase in amputation risk, and a comprehensive analysis of the CANVAS program failed to identify any baseline characteristics that increased an individual's risk of amputation with canagliflozin therapy. This included systolic blood pressure and body mass index (BMI), as well as concomitant use of diuretics or other antihypertensive therapies.[19] Furthermore, given that diuresis, natriuresis, reduction in blood pressure and lowering of body weight are class effects of SGLT2 inhibitors, and not specific to canagliflozin, if these factors do precipitate an increase in amputation risk it should have been seen with all compounds in the class. A second possible causal mechanism based on "hemoconcentration" was also widely considered–SGLT2 inhibitors increase hematocrit, and it was proposed that this may be sufficient to impede the circulation in serious peripheral artery disease.[19,29] Once again, however, hemoconcentration is a feature of all SGLT2 inhibitors, and this mechanism is unable to explain the absence of amputation risk across other drugs in the class. This mechanism was explored in an animal study that used a hindlimb ischemia model in mice to test the hypothesis that canagliflozin impairs limb blood flow secondary to hemoconcentration, particularly in the presence of peripheral arterial disease. That study showed no effect of canagliflozin on the recovery of perfusion or vascular recovery.[30]

More challenging still to efforts to define a mechanism of causation is the observation that the adverse effects of canagliflozin on amputation risk were observed in the CANVAS program but not the CREDENCE trial, both of which investigated the effects canagliflozin. With this discrepancy making it unlikely that it is a drug specific effect of canagliflozin, and trials of other agents having tested SGLT2 inhibition in the CANVAS and CREDENCE population groups with no evidence of an increased risk, chance may be the most plausible explanation for the CANVAS program amputation result. Reflecting the accumulating data about amputation, the null CREDENCE trial findings and the absence of amputation risk with any other SGLT2 inhibitor, in 2020, the FDA "boxed warning" for amputation was removed from canagliflozin.

FRACTURE
Canagliflozin and Fracture Risk

An increase in fracture with SGLT2 inhibitor treatment was also first identified in the CANVAS program during an interim review of data by the Independent Data Monitoring Committee.[4] In a population of T2D patients, 4.9% had a fracture during follow-up, with canagliflozin increasing the risk of fracture by 26% (HR 1.26; 95% CI 1.04, 1.52). The effects of canagliflozin for this outcome seemed consistent across participant subgroups defined by age, sex, race, BMI, comorbidities and medication use. However, the CANVAS program comprised 2 component studies, CANVAS and CANVAS-R, and there was significant heterogeneity (p interaction = 0.005) between the 55% increase in fracture risk observed in CANVAS (HR 1.55; 95% CI 1.21, 1.97) and the null effect on fracture observed in CANVAS-R (HR 0.86; 95% CI 0.62, 1.19). An in-depth analysis explored multiple possible explanations for the different findings across the 2 studies including participant characteristics, doses of randomized treatment, durations of follow-up and the occurrence of falls

during the trials.[31] Ultimately, it proved impossible to identify a mechanism to explain the differences based on biology, trial features, or patient characteristics, and it was concluded that chance was the most likely explanation for the observed adverse effect in CANVAS. Subsequently, the CREDENCE trial, which also evaluated the effect of canagliflozin, reported no increase in fracture risk with canagliflozin treatment (HR 0.98, 95% CI 0.70, 1.37)[7] providing some further support for chance as the explanation.

All sodium glucose cotransporter 2 inhibitors and fracture risk

Across the 11 large randomized clinical trials of this drug class, there has only been an adverse fracture risk observed in the CANVAS program, with no significant increase in fracture identified in any of the other studies (**Fig. 3**A). Meta-analysis done for this report to explore fracture risk by study population showed no evidence of increased fracture in those with T2D (RR 1.06; 95% CI 0.97, 1.15), CKD (RR 1.03; 95% CI 0.87, 1.22), or heart failure (RR 1.06; 95% CI 0.89, 1.27) with broadly consistent sets of findings for each set of trials (all p heterogeneity > 0.441) (**Fig. 3**B). Visual examination of the forest plots for fracture risk, as for amputation outcomes, identifies the CANVAS program result as an outlier.

Potential mechanisms for causation of fracture with sodium glucose cotransporter 2 inhibition

Patients with T2D are known to be at an elevated risk of fracture due to changes in bone architecture and bone composition with evidence of decreased bone turnover, although no reduction in bone mineral density. Older age and obesity further exacerbate fracture risk in this population,[32] which is also at elevated risk of falling due to neuropathy, retinopathy, balance, and strength. Those with CKD are another high-risk population with an increased risk of developing bone mineral disorders and fractures.[33] Rates of fracture were therefore anticipated to be high for most trials of SGLT2 inhibitors, but there was no a priori expectation that SGLT2 inhibitor therapy would either increase or decrease fracture risk.

The reported adverse effect of canagliflozin on fracture in CANVAS resulted in extensive investigation and careful consideration of diverse possible causal mechanisms. Canagliflozin, and SGLT2 inhibitors more broadly, do not change serum calcium, vitamin D, or parathyroid

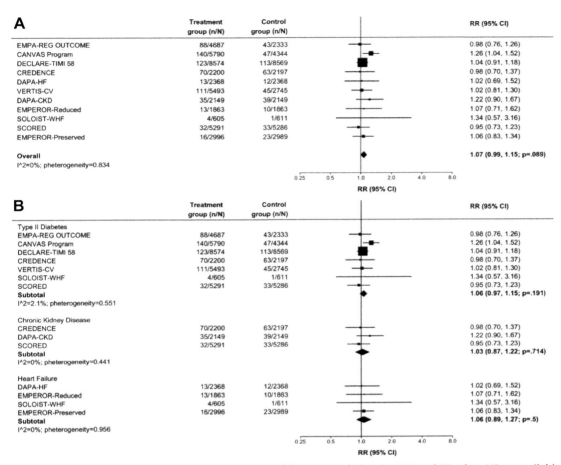

Fig. 3. Fracture Risk Overall (*A*) and by Trial Population (*B*). Meta-analysis using HR and RR when HR unavailable performed using random-effects meta-analysis using R. HR used: CANVAS, DECLARE-TIMI 58, CREDENCE. RR used: EMPA-REG Outcome, DAPA-HF, VERTIS-CV, DAPA-CKD, EMPEROR-Reduced, SOLOIST-WHF, SCORED, EMPEROR-Preserved.

hormone and effects on serum phosphate and magnesium are only small. One report identified a possible effect of canagliflozin on markers of bone turnover and another showed small changes in bone mineral density, although this latter observation was inconsistent across the skeletal sites measured and was of a magnitude consistent with the weight loss effects achieved in the trial.[34] There was no bone metabolism effect of canagliflozin identified that was able to explain the large increase in risk observed in CANVAS and, as for amputation, the inconsistency in findings across CANVAS, CANVAS-R and CREDENCE made a drug-specific explanation unlikely–true effects of canagliflozin observed in CANVAS should have been replicated in CANVAS-R and CREDENCE.

The other widely cited possible reason for an increased fracture risk with canagliflozin was an increased rate of falls in the intervention group

caused by volume depletion, blood pressure lowering, and episodes of hypotension. Falls were not systematically recorded in the CANVAS program, so the depth of possible analysis was limited, but the investigation of the adverse event records identified no increase in falls.[31] Further, if this were the mechanism of action for an increased fracture risk, the same signal would have been anticipated in CANVAS-R and CREDENCE as well as all the other SGLT2 trials, and this was not observed. Similarly, the T2D population studied in CANVAS has been the subject of many other trials of SGLT2 inhibition with no evidence that this population subset is at risk of fracture when exposed to SGLT2 inhibition. In the absence of any plausible mechanism being identified, and given the solitary nature of the fracture finding in just one trial, the most likely explanation for the fracture risk observed in CANVAS seems to be chance.

SGLT2 Inhibitors

| Broad cardiovascular and renal benefits in those with T2D, CKD and heart failure |

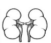

Amputation

No increase in RR of amputation:
- Overall
- By individual drug
- By patient population

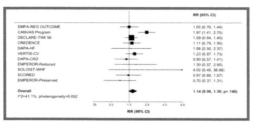

Fracture

No increase in RR of fracture:
- Overall
- By individual drug
- By patient population

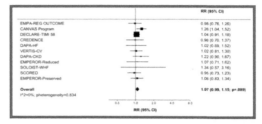

Fig. 4. Central figure- SGLT2 inhibitors: amputation and fracture risk. CKD, chronic kidney disease; RR, relative risk; SGLT2inhibitor, sodium glucose cotransporter 2 inhibitor; T2D, type 2 diabetes.

CHANCE FINDINGS IN LARGE-SCALE TRIALS

In this review, we have concluded that the increased risks of amputation and fracture reported for the SGLT2 inhibitor canagliflozin were both likely to have arisen by chance. These conclusions are based primarily on the observations that the effects were reported in single studies, there was no coherence of findings across similar studies, and despite intensive investigation, no plausible causal mechanism could be identified.

Concluding chance findings from large-scale trials is an uncomfortable and somewhat counterintuitive act. Well-conducted large-scale trials are designed specifically to detect the plausible effects of an intervention and to protect against chance findings. However, that is only strictly true for those outcomes that are the prespecified objectives of the study, for which the sample size has been selected and the analysis strategy planned. By contrast, the amputation and fracture risks identified for canagliflozin were entirely unexpected observations that resulted from serial analyses done by the Independent Data Monitoring Committee to ensure the safety of trial participants taking a new drug class. Although members of Independent Data Monitoring Committees are careful to consider the potential impact of multiple analyses of data, the process inevitably increases the likelihood that false-positive findings will arise.

Serial analyses of data for safety monitoring can produce spurious findings in just the same way that post hoc analyses of exploratory outcomes and effects in participants subgroups can produce unexpected observations. Doing more analyses increases the likelihood that something will arise by chance. For investigations of novel drug therapies, serial monitoring is an essential part of the business of ensuring participant safety. However, even when done to a high standard by high-quality technicians, it is not without potential adverse consequences. Canagliflozin was suspected for many years to cause an increased risk of fracture and amputation based on findings that now seem to be the result of chance. These CANVAS program findings required enormous effort to fully understand their implications and have had major impacts of the perceived safety of SGLT2 inhibitors in general, and canagliflozin in particular. Only with multiple studies of canagliflozin and many subsequent trials of other SGLT2 inhibitors done over a prolonged period, has it been possible to infer the most likely effects of SGLT2 inhibitors on these risks.

SUMMARY

SGLT2 inhibitors are associated with clear CV and renal benefits across a broad spectrum of patients, with no increase in total serious adverse events. The available data make it unlikely that canagliflozin, or SGLT2 inhibitors more broadly, increase the risk of amputation or fracture either overall or in any specific population subset. The increased amputation and fracture risks with canagliflozin treatment identified in the CANVAS program seem most likely to have been chance findings (**Fig. 4**).

CLINICS CARE POINTS

> - Patients with type 2 diabetes (T2D) and chronic kidney disease (CKD) are at elevated risk of amputation and fracture.
> - Treatment with sodium glucose cotransporter 2 (SGLT2) inhibitors does not increase the risk of amputation or fracture overall or in any patients group defined by their comorbidities or demographics.
> - Given the significant cardiovascular and renal benefits of SGLT2 inhibitors, they should be considered in all eligible patients with T2D, CKD, or heart failure.
> - Close attention should be paid to bone health, falls risk, and limb care in these populations, but concerns about fracture risk and amputation are not a reason for withholding SGLT2 inhibitor therapy.

DISCLOSURE

A/Professor C. Arnott is involved in the secondary analysis program for the CANVAS program and CREDENCE trials at the George Institute for Global Health. Mr R.A. Fletcher has no disclosures. Professor B. Neal has received grants for CANVAS and CREDENCE, Advisory Board, Honoraria, Travel reimbursement all from Janssen and all paid to his institution.

REFERENCES

1. American Diabetes A. 8. Pharmacologic approaches to glycemic treatment: standards of medical care in diabetes-2018. Diabetes Care 2018; 41(Suppl 1):S73–85.
2. American Diabetes A. 1. Improving care and promoting health in populations: standards of medical care in diabetes-2019. Diabetes Care 2019; 42(Suppl 1):S7–12.
3. Garber AJ, Abrahamson MJ, Barzilay JI, et al. Consensus statement by the american association of clinical endocrinologists and american college of endocrinology on the comprehensive type 2 diabetes management algorithm - 2018 executive summary. Endocr Pract 2018;24(1):91–120.
4. Neal B, Perkovic V, Matthews DR. Canagliflozin and cardiovascular and renal events in type 2 diabetes. N Engl J Med 2017;377(21):2099.
5. Wiviott SD, Raz I, Bonaca MP, et al. Dapagliflozin and cardiovascular outcomes in type 2 diabetes. N Engl J Med 2018;10. https://doi.org/10.1056/NEJMoa1812389.
6. Zinman B, Wanner C, Lachin JM, et al. Empagliflozin, cardiovascular outcomes, and mortality in type 2 diabetes. N Engl J Med 2015;373(22): 2117–28.
7. Perkovic V, Jardine MJ, Neal B, et al. Canagliflozin and renal outcomes in type 2 diabetes and nephropathy. N Engl J Med 2019. https://doi.org/10.1056/NEJMoa1811744.
8. Arnott C, Li Q, Kang A, et al. Sodium-glucose cotransporter 2 inhibition for the prevention of cardiovascular events in patients with type 2 diabetes mellitus: a systematic review and meta-analysis. J Am Heart Assoc 2020;9(3):e014908.
9. Neuen BL, Young T, Heerspink HJL, et al. SGLT2 inhibitors for the prevention of kidney failure in patients with type 2 diabetes: a systematic review and meta-analysis. Lancet Diabetes Endocrinol 2019;7(11):845–54.
10. Heerspink HJL, Stefansson BV, Correa-Rotter R, et al. Dapagliflozin in patients with chronic kidney disease. N Engl J Med 2020;383(15):1436–46.
11. McMurray JJV, Solomon SD, Inzucchi SE, et al. Dapagliflozin in patients with heart failure and reduced ejection fraction. N Engl J Med 2019;381(21): 1995–2008.
12. Packer M, Anker SD, Butler J, et al. Cardiovascular and renal outcomes with empagliflozin in heart failure. N Engl J Med 2020;383(15):1413–24.
13. Anker SD, Butler J, Filippatos G, et al. Empagliflozin in heart failure with a preserved ejection fraction. N Engl J Med 2021;385(16):1451–61.
14. Yu J, Zhou Z, Mahaffey KW, et al. An exploration of the heterogeneity in effects of SGLT2 inhibition on cardiovascular and all-cause mortality in the EMPA-REG OUTCOME, CANVAS Program, DECLARE-TIMI 58, and CREDENCE trials. Int J Cardiol 2021;324:165–72.
15. Zelniker TA, Wiviott SD, Raz I, et al. SGLT2 inhibitors for primary and secondary prevention of cardiovascular and renal outcomes in type 2 diabetes: a systematic review and meta-analysis of cardiovascular outcome trials. Lancet 2019;393(10166):31–9.
16. American Diabetes A. 10. Cardiovascular disease and risk management: standards of medical care in diabetes-2020. Diabetes Care 2020;43(Suppl 1): S111–34.
17. McDonagh TA, Metra M, Adamo M, et al. 2021 ESC Guidelines for the diagnosis and treatment of acute and chronic heart failure. Eur Heart J 2021;42(36): 3599–726.
18. Jeong SJ, Lee SE, Shin DH, et al. Barriers to initiating SGLT2 inhibitors in diabetic kidney disease: a real-world study. BMC Nephrol 2021;22(1):177.
19. Arnott C, Huang Y, Neuen BL, et al. The effect of canagliflozin on amputation risk in the CANVAS program and the CREDENCE trial. Diabetes Obes Metab 2020;22(10):1753–66.

20. Udell JA, Yuan Z, Rush T, et al. Cardiovascular outcomes and risks after initiation of a sodium glucose cotransporter 2 inhibitor: results from the EASEL population-based cohort study (evidence for cardiovascular outcomes with sodium glucose cotransporter 2 inhibitors in the real world). Circulation 2018;137(14):1450–9.

21. Fralick M, Kim SC, Schneeweiss S, et al. Risk of amputation with canagliflozin across categories of age and cardiovascular risk in three US nationwide databases: cohort study. BMJ 2020;370:m2812.

22. Ryan PB, Buse JB, Schuemie MJ, et al. Comparative effectiveness of canagliflozin, SGLT2 inhibitors and non-SGLT2 inhibitors on the risk of hospitalization for heart failure and amputation in patients with type 2 diabetes mellitus: a real-world meta-analysis of 4 observational databases (OBSERVE-4D). Diabetes Obes Metab 2018;20(11):2585–97.

23. Paul SK, Bhatt DL, Montvida O. The association of amputations and peripheral artery disease in patients with type 2 diabetes mellitus receiving sodium-glucose cotransporter type-2 inhibitors: real-world study. Eur Heart J 2021;42(18):1728–38.

24. Bhatt DL, Szarek M, Pitt B, et al. Sotagliflozin in patients with diabetes and chronic kidney disease. N Engl J Med 2021;384(2):129–39.

25. Bhatt DL, Szarek M, Steg PG, et al. Sotagliflozin in patients with diabetes and recent worsening heart failure. N Engl J Med 2021;384(2):117–28.

26. Cannon CP, Pratley R, Dagogo-Jack S, et al. Cardiovascular Outcomes with Ertugliflozin in Type 2 diabetes. N Engl J Med 2020;383(15):1425–35.

27. Barnes JA, Eid MA, Creager MA, et al. Epidemiology and risk of amputation in patients with diabetes mellitus and peripheral artery disease. Arterioscler Thromb Vasc Biol 2020;40(8):1808–17.

28. Lin C, Zhu X, Cai X, et al. SGLT2 inhibitors and lower limb complications: an updated meta-analysis. Cardiovasc Diabetol 2021;20(1):91.

29. Potier L, Roussel R, Velho G, et al. Lower limb events in individuals with type 2 diabetes: evidence for an increased risk associated with diuretic use. Diabetologia 2019;62(6):939–47.

30. Sherman SE, Bell GI, Teoh H, et al. Canagliflozin improves the recovery of blood flow in an experimental model of severe limb ischemia. JACC Basic Transl Sci 2018;3(2):327–9.

31. Zhou Z, Jardine M, Perkovic V, et al. Canagliflozin and fracture risk in individuals with type 2 diabetes: results from the CANVAS program. Diabetologia 2019;62(10):1854–67.

32. Leslie WD, Rubin MR, Schwartz AV, et al. Type 2 diabetes and bone. J Bone Miner Res 2012;27(11):2231–7.

33. Torres PAU, Cohen-Solal M. Evaluation of fracture risk in chronic kidney disease. J Nephrol 2017;30(5):653–61.

34. Blevins TC, Farooki A. Bone effects of canagliflozin, a sodium glucose co-transporter 2 inhibitor, in patients with type 2 diabetes mellitus. Postgrad Med 2017;129(1):159–68.

UNITED STATES POSTAL SERVICE ®

Statement of Ownership, Management, and Circulation
(All Periodicals Publications Except Requester Publications)

1. Publication Title	2. Publication Number	3. Filing Date
HEART FAILURE CLINICS	025 – 055	9/18/2022

4. Issue Frequency	5. Number of Issues Published Annually	6. Annual Subscription Price
JAN, APR, JUL, OCT	4	$277.00

7. Complete Mailing Address of Known Office of Publication *(Not printer) (Street, city, county, state, and ZIP+4®)*

ELSEVIER INC.
230 Park Avenue, Suite 800
New York, NY 10169

Contact Person
Malathi Samayan

Telephone *(Include area code)*
91-44-4299-4507

8. Complete Mailing Address of Headquarters or General Business Office of Publisher *(Not printer)*

ELSEVIER INC.
230 Park Avenue, Suite 800
New York, NY 10169

9. Full Names and Complete Mailing Addresses of Publisher, Editor, and Managing Editor *(Do not leave blank)*

Publisher *(Name and complete mailing address)*

Dolores Meloni, ELSEVIER INC.
1600 JOHN F KENNEDY BLVD. SUITE 1800
PHILADELPHIA, PA 19103-2899

Editor *(Name and complete mailing address)*

JOANNA COLLETT, ELSEVIER INC.
1600 JOHN F KENNEDY BLVD. SUITE 1800
PHILADELPHIA, PA 19103-2899

Managing Editor *(Name and complete mailing address)*

PATRICK MANLEY, ELSEVIER INC.
1600 JOHN F KENNEDY BLVD. SUITE 1800
PHILADELPHIA, PA 19103-2899

10. Owner *(Do not leave blank. If the publication is owned by a corporation, give the name and address of the corporation immediately followed by the names and addresses of all stockholders owning or holding 1 percent or more of the total amount of stock. If not owned by a corporation, give the names and addresses of the individual owners. If owned by a partnership or other unincorporated firm, give its name and address as well as those of each individual owner. If the publication is published by a nonprofit organization, give its name and address.)*

Full Name	Complete Mailing Address
	1600 JOHN F KENNEDY BLVD. SUITE 1800 PHILADELPHIA, PA 19103-2899
WHOLLY OWNED SUBSIDIARY OF REED/ELSEVIER, US HOLDINGS	

11. Known Bondholders, Mortgagees, and Other Security Holders Owning or Holding 1 Percent or More of Total Amount of Bonds, Mortgages, or Other Securities. If none, check box ▶ ☐ None

Full Name	Complete Mailing Address
N/A	

12. Tax Status *(For completion by nonprofit organizations authorized to mail at nonprofit rates) (Check one)*
The purpose, function, and nonprofit status of this organization and the exempt status for federal income tax purposes:
☒ Has Not Changed During Preceding 12 Months
☐ Has Changed During Preceding 12 Months *(Publisher must submit explanation of change with this statement)*

PS Form **3526**, July 2014 *[Page 1 of 4 (see instructions page 4)]* PSN: 7530-01-000-9931   PRIVACY NOTICE: See our privacy policy on www.usps.com.

---

13. Publication Title	14. Issue Date for Circulation Data Below
HEART FAILURE CLINICS	JULY 2022

15. Extent and Nature of Circulation			Average No. Copies Each Issue During Preceding 12 Months	No. Copies of Single Issue Published Nearest to Filing Date
a. Total Number of Copies *(Net press run)*			36	31
b. Paid Circulation (By Mail and Outside the Mail)	(1)	Mailed Outside-County Paid Subscriptions Stated on PS Form 3541 (Include paid distribution above nominal rate, advertiser's proof copies, and exchange copies)	18	16
	(2)	Mailed In-County Paid Subscriptions Stated on PS Form 3541 (Include paid distribution above nominal rate, advertiser's proof copies, and exchange copies)	0	0
	(3)	Paid Distribution Outside the Mails Including Sales Through Dealers and Carriers, Street Vendors, Counter Sales, and Other Paid Distribution Outside USPS®	10	9
	(4)	Paid Distribution by Other Classes of Mail Through the USPS (e.g., First-Class Mail®)	0	0
c. Total Paid Distribution *(Sum of 15b (1), (2), (3), and (4))*		▶	28	25
d. Free or Nominal Rate Distribution (By Mail and Outside the Mail)	(1)	Free or Nominal Rate Outside-County Copies included on PS Form 3541	8	6
	(2)	Free or Nominal Rate In-County Copies Included on PS Form 3541	0	0
	(3)	Free or Nominal Rate Copies Mailed at Other Classes Through the USPS (e.g. First-Class Mail)	0	0
	(4)	Free or Nominal Rate Distribution Outside the Mail (Carriers or other means)	0	0
e. Total Free or Nominal Rate Distribution *(Sum of 15d (1), (2), (3) and (4))*		▶	8	6
f. Total Distribution *(Sum of 15c and 15e)*		▶	36	31
g. Copies not Distributed *(See Instructions to Publishers #4 (page #3))*		▶	0	0
h. Total *(Sum of 15f and g)*		▶	36	31
i. Percent Paid *(15c divided by 15f times 100)*			77.77%	80.64%

If you are claiming electronic copies go to line 16 on page 3. If you are not claiming electronic copies, skip to line 17 on page 3.

PS Form **3526**, July 2014 (Page 2 of 4)

16. Electronic Copy Circulation	Average No. Copies Each Issue During Preceding 12 Months	No. Copies of Single Issue Published Nearest to Filing Date
a. Paid Electronic Copies ▶		
b. Total Paid Print Copies (Line 15c) + Paid Electronic Copies (Line 16a) ▶		
c. Total Print Distribution (Line 15f) + Paid Electronic Copies (Line 16a) ▶		
d. Percent Paid (Both Print & Electronic Copies) (16b divided by 16c × 100) ▶		

☒ I certify that 50% of all my distributed copies (electronic and print) are paid above a nominal price.

17. Publication of Statement of Ownership

☒ If the publication is a general publication, publication of this statement is required. Will be printed in the **OCTOBER 2022** issue of this publication.   ☐ Publication not required.

18. Signature and Title of Editor, Publisher, Business Manager, or Owner

Malathi Samayan

Malathi Samayan - Distribution Controller   Date 9/18/2022

I certify that all information furnished on this form is true and complete. I understand that anyone who furnishes false or misleading information on this form or who omits material or information requested on the form may be subject to criminal sanctions (including fines and imprisonment) and/or civil sanctions (including civil penalties).

PS Form **3526**, July 2014 (Page 3 of 4)   PRIVACY NOTICE: See our privacy policy on www.usps.com

Moving?

Make sure your subscription moves with you!

To notify us of your new address, find your **Clinics Account Number** (located on your mailing label above your name), and contact customer service at:

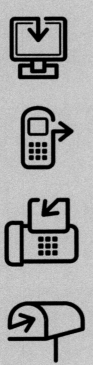

Email: journalscustomerservice-usa@elsevier.com

800-654-2452 (subscribers in the U.S. & Canada)
314-447-8871 (subscribers outside of the U.S. & Canada)

Fax number: 314-447-8029

Elsevier Health Sciences Division
Subscription Customer Service
3251 Riverport Lane
Maryland Heights, MO 63043

ELSEVIER